Aging
and
Prevention
New Approaches for Preventing Health and Mental Health Problems in Older Adults

The *Prevention in Human Services* series:

Aging
and
Prevention

New Approaches for Preventing Health and Mental Health Problems in Older Adults

Edited by
Sharon Simson, Laura B. Wilson,
Jared Hermalin, and Robert Hess

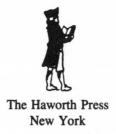

The Haworth Press
New York

Aging and Prevention: New Approaches for Preventing Health and Mental Health Problems in Older Adults has also been published as *Prevention in Human Services,* Volume 3, Number 1, Fall 1983.

The Haworth Press, Inc., 28 East 22 Street, New York, NY 10010

Library of Congress Cataloging in Publication Data
Main entry under title:

Aging and prevention.

   "Has also been published as Prevention in human services, volume 3, number 1, fall 1983."—T.p. verso.
   Includes bibliographical references.
   1. Geriatrics. 2. Medicine, Preventive. 3. Gerontology. I. Simson, Sharon. [DNLM: 1. Aging. 2. Community mental health services—In old age. 3. Health services for the aged. 4. Preventive health services. W1 PR497 v. 3 no. 1/WT 30 A2675]
RC952.5.A435 1983   613'.0438   83-17172
ISBN 0-86656-188-9

Aging and Prevention
New Approaches for Preventing Health and Mental Health Problems in Older Adults

Prevention in Human Services
Volume 3, Number 1

CONTENTS

Aging
and
Prevention
New Approaches for Preventing Health and Mental Health Problems in Older Adults

Preface

The development of prevention programs for older Americans has not received sufficient attention in the literature. Indeed, prevention has traditionally been associated with the younger age cohorts of our society: the infant, toddler, early child (ages 5–8), middle child (ages 9–12), pre-adolescent, and adolescent. We have neglected our older societal members who, with advancing age, need our help that much more.

Given an increasingly older population, it becomes imperative that we question the priority ratings assigned to various target age cohorts. In doing so, we necessarily call into examination our values, norms, standards, and traditions.

To illustrate, older members of American society have traditionally not been held in high esteem. They have stereotypically been viewed as non-productive members of a work-oriented economy, a burden on their families, and a drain on societal resources. As a result, we have frequently paid greater heed to the needs of our younger age groups, who it is thought can provide greater future potential to family, community, and economy.

Closer examination reveals, however, that many legislators, judges, corporate board members, and community leaders have contributed much beyond their 65th birthdays. Indeed, many older workers are requesting that their jobs be maintained beyond the specified retirement age.

Given more comprehensive prevention programs targeted toward older Americans, the range of contributions can be substantial. From a cost-benefit perspective, a more healthy, industrious older population would also result in sizeable reductions in medical and hospital expenses, welfare costs, and social security payments, while at the same time contributing to an increased gross national product and standard of living. Observed from a sociopsychological perspective, prevention programs would be quite useful in enhancing one's self-esteem, sense of worth, and vitality, while reducing the prevalence of depression and suicidal ideation, problems all too common among the older adult population.

1

In short, raising the issue of prevention programs for the elderly involves a potential savings of millions of dollars, in addition to the sanctity of an individual's right to live out his or her remaining days in relative peace and comfort. It is thus necessary that we review our funding priorities and cultural norms and values, so that we may be better equipped to deal with an ever increasing older population, a population which one day will include us.

Jared Hermalin
Robert Hess

Introduction

In the past twenty years the delivery of health services to the elderly population has been profoundly impacted upon by a number of factors: technological advances in science, medicine, and nutrition; a longer life span; increased vulnerability to chronic illnesses and environmental hazards; and changing cultural roles and responsibilities (Association of American Medical Colleges Task Force on Graduate Medical Education, 1981; Sherwood, 1975). By the year 2000, 12% of the population will be over 65 (U.S. Senate, 1982). Illness rates, disability rates, hospital utilization, number of physician visits, and chronic ailments all increase sharply with age (Brody, 1979). Persons over age 65 account for 30% of total personal health care expenditures and their medical costs are approximately three times greater than those under 65 (Moore, Friedman, & Warshaw, 1981).

One feasible response to the growing needs of the elderly is to expand the scope of health care services, research, and education and training from an acute focus to include an emphasis on preventive measures which impact upon the aging process and the noncurative, multifaceted, long term care needs associated with chronic diseases (Anderson, 1978; German, 1981). This position has been advanced by the Office of Disease Prevention and Health Promotion in *Prevention '80* (U.S. Department of Health and Human Services, 1980).

Although prevention has become a familiar concept which has been used in research, education, and practice related to younger populations, the application of "prevention" to aging is an unusual and novel idea. This collection of papers provides a starting point for exploring various meanings of prevention and the significance of prevention activities to one particular age cohort, the elderly.

"Social Policies and Programs for the Elderly as Mechanisms of Prevention," by Lowy defines the concept of prevention and discusses the three stages in the process of prevention. This conceptual material serves as a foundation for the consideration of two key issues related to the elderly: (1) social policies as mechanisms of primary prevention, and (2) social/mental health services as mechanisms of secondary and tertiary prevention. Practical information about numerous programs and services is brought together and presented in a systematic, useful way.

"The Status of Preventive Care for the Aged: A Meta-Analysis," by Wilson, Simson, and McCaughey identifies and reviews research and programmatic activities which have been reported in the literature during the last ten years in the area of prevention and aging. An evaluation process, meta-analysis, is used to assess the therapeutic effect and overall effectiveness of techniques in prevention and aging. The paper considers expansion of the definition and scope of preventive care from the younger and middle age cohorts to include an emphasis on preventive care for older people.

"Healthy Aging Through Knowledge and Self Care," by Gioiella examines changes related to normal aging and health maintenance behaviors. Changes covered are physical, sensory, mobility, tissue, psychosocial, and sexuality. Services needed to support health maintenance are discussed including teaching and counseling, screening/referral, and activity oriented services.

"Targeting Community Services to High-Risk Elders: Toward Preventing Long-Term Care Institutionalization," by Jette and Branch addresses three prevention questions: (1) can risk factors for long term care institutionalization be identified empirically; (2) can home care be targeted to high risk groups; and (3) does targeting services in this manner prevent long term care institutionalization?

"An Alternative Health Delivery System for the Chronically Ill Elderly," by Weiss and Sklar presents an innovative alternative delivery system, Project Open. Project Open is designed to provide preventive health and social services in order to reduce costs and provide more effective care. A time series experimental method is used to study Project Open participants. Findings indicate a maintenance in functioning levels of Project Open participants, a decrease in acute hospitalization, and a reduction in health care costs.

"Prevention of Unnecessary Geriatric Deaths: Differential Rates of Morbidity/Mortality on Admission to Long Term Care Facilities," by West assesses rates of morbidity and mortality associated with institutionalization. Implications for timely and appropriate intervention at the time of institutionalization are considered, particularly in terms of naturally occurring phenomena.

"Health, Prevention and Televison: Images of the Elderly and Perception of Social Reality," by Signorielli presents findings from a fourteen year Cultural Indicators research project that included an examination of the relationship between television, aging, health, and prevention. This study focuses on the presentation of older characters and old age in prime time network television drama with special attention to what these images reveal about aging, health, and prevention.

"Opportunities for Prevention of Domestic Neglect and Abuse of the Elderly," by Douglass reports that the target group of highest risk is the oldest and most frail elderly. The study suggests that neglect and abuse can be ameliorated through primary prevention activities conducted by a system of mental health, public health, and social services.

"Older Women and Informal Supports: Impact on Prevention," by Quam reports on a study of the nature, quality, functions, and use of friends by older women. The ways in which friends can function in preventive ways are explored and suggestions are offered regarding the design of programs to maximize interaction among older women and other informal supports.

These studies explore various aspects of aging and prevention. When taken together, they provide a foundation to aid others in their quest for a more realistic, modern day version of the fountain of youth.

Sharon Simson
Laura B. Wilson

REFERENCES

Anderson, F. Preventive medicine in old age. In J.C. Brocklehurst (Ed.), *Textbook of Geriatric medicine and gerontology.* London: Churchill Livingstone, 1978.

Association of American Medical Colleges Task Force on Graduate Medical Education. Proposals for the eighties. *Journal of Medical Education,* 1981, *56*(9), Part 2.

Brody, E. M. Long term care for the aged: Promises and prospects. *Health and Social Work,* 1979, *4*(1), 29.

German, P. S. Delivery of care to older people: Issues and outlooks. *Topics in Clinical Nursing,* 1981, *3*(1), 1–13.

Moore, J. T., Friedman, S. S., & Warshaw, G. A. Geriatric medicine training in a family medicine residency. *Journal of Medical Education,* 1981, *56*(6), 492–496.

Sherwood, S. (Ed.) *Long-term care: A handbook for researchers, planners, and providers.* New York: Halsted Press, 1975.

U.S. Department of Health and Human Services, Public Health Service, Office of Disease Prevention and Health Promotion. *Prevention '80* (Publication No. 81-50157). Washington, DC: U.S. Government Printing Office, 1980.

U.S. Senate, Special Committee on Aging. *Every ninth American.* Washington, DC: U.S. Government Printing Office, 1982.

Social Policies and Programs for the Elderly as Mechanisms of Prevention

Louis Lowy

ABSTRACT. The concept of prevention is defined and the role of social policy as a primary prevention mechanism is explored. Common programs for the elderly and their strengths and limitations are described. Recommendations are made for new social policies, based on the philosophy of prevention, which are comprehensive, flexible, responsive, and informed by the elderly themselves.

There are more elderly people in our society today than ever before. Many are independent, vigorous and flourishing. But there are also more at-risk older people today than ever before. The problems they face cannot be neatly divided into the physical, the mental, the social, and the financial. It is often a constellation of stresses and deprivations that threaten the well-being and survival of the vulnerable old person. During the normal aging process, natural life crises such as the loss of family and friends and the resulting loss of social supports, the fear of death, dying, and invalidism, and increased social isolation and physical disability can contribute to an elderly person being at risk of developing mental health problems requiring treatment and other services (Bengtson & Treas, 1980; Kirschner, 1979; Miller, 1981).

Often a major crisis involves the loss of physical capacities and the resulting inability of an elderly person to remain independently in his/her own home. Frequently, the pressures for placing such an individual in a nursing home or total care environment supersede a careful approach to selecting other alternatives that would allow the aged person to remain at home or move to a less than total environ-

Reprints may be requested from Louis Lowy, School of Social Work, Boston University, 264 Bay State Road, Boston, MA 02215.

7

ment. But all too often there are no alternatives available (Brody, 1979).

The process of aging corresponds to a complex set of interrelated biological, psychological, and sociological forces which interact and affect the nature and quality of human development in later life. It is important to understand the aging experience as a dynamic interplay of inputs from a multiplicity of sources. Aging is not experienced in the same manner by all members of society; it is subject to the same diversity and differentiations found in other stages of the life cycle.

Concept of Prevention

In its rudimentary sense, "prevention" simply means keeping something from happening. Beyond that simple definition, the term has taken on multiple connotations. Society tries to "prevent" all kinds of things—accidents, crime, diseases, wars. With respect to social problems, the idea of prevention is not new. In 1818, the Society for the Prevention of Pauperism was formed to stamp out the "pestilence of pauperism," along with crime and delinquency, and in 1874, the Society for the Prevention of Cruelty to Children came into being.

Key concepts include the identification of stages in the process of prevention. *Primary prevention* refers to elimination of the problem at its source, procedures that make a "population at-risk" invulnerable to it. *Secondary prevention* involves efforts to curtail the spread of the problems to others and to interrupt its course. *Tertiary prevention* aims to reduce the duration and severity of disabling sequelae (Giovannoni, 1982).

During the later years of life, problems arise as a result of the interface between unmet personal needs and situational and environmental difficulties and insufficiencies. The effects on older people are differential, depending on variables such as personality, sex, class position, cultural background, race, and ethnicity. Older people in general are defined as a "population-at-risk." Among older people, especially those in the later years, there are persons (the frail elderly) who are even more vulnerable to debilitating conditions in their immediate environment, who have greater physical and emotional disabilities than their contemporaries, whose functional and coping abilities are more severely impaired and who are, therefore, more dependent on psychological, physical, and social measures than other aging persons. In the majority of these cases, prevention can be tertiary at best, and stop-gap support measures as well as caring functions are the predominant "treatment of choice" interventions.

Social Policies as Mechanisms of Primary Prevention

Social policies have been developed as mechanisms of primary prevention which are designed to eliminate the problem at its source. Since the later years pose natural risks to income, health, and physical and social living arrangements, primary prevention is to be geared to insure protection against such risk conditions (Estes, 1979).

Income. The Social Security program is a major bulwark against income loss and provides an income floor based on the assumption of earned right. Economic support of an older population is a fiscal and a political matter. The combination of demographic, economic, and employment trends can seriously threaten both the elderly's income security and the financial viability of government support programs. Although the present income structure, consisting of social security, pensions, savings, and sporadic employment, has reduced poverty among the elderly, poverty is still disproportionately high. Moreover, the present economic structure makes it unlikely that during the later years of life and aged person will be able to maintain a standard of living equivalent to that enjoyed earlier in life. Although it is true that persons retiring today are relatively better off than their predecessors, mandatory and even voluntary retirement for many persons still significantly increases the probability of severe income loss, decline in living standard, and impoverishment. Elderly women—mostly widows—are particular victims of poverty due to inequities in income maintenance provisions such as social security and pensions. This development occurs against the backdrop of a recognition on the part of public policymakers that the financing of the Social Security Act must be rethought and rearranged, as is evident in the laws passed by Congress during the Spring of 1983.

Supplementary Security Income (SSI), private and public pension benefits, food stamps, and tax benefits are geared to prevent outright poverty and destitution, despite their shortcomings. However, it must be noted that income conditions of older persons are always related to the economic conditions of the country. The rate of economic growth, inflation, unemployment, allocation of the economic pie based on societal values, support for competing economic claims, and moves toward reducing inequality for the total population are the powerful variables that affect any income policy as a mechanism of primary prevention for the elderly.

Health. Primary prevention in health and mental health of the elderly is based on a definition of health which is determined by level of functioning. "Health in the elderly is best measured in terms of function. . .degree of fitness rather than extent of pathology may be used as a measure of the amount of services the aged will require from the community" (Lowy, 1980). Health is not a matter of the elderly's access to treatment for specific illnesses, but also a question of how a full array of health-related services can help them remain in the best possible physical and mental health in order to stay in the mainstream of community life. This means that sufficient societal resources have to be secured for nutrition, health education, and biomedical research to cope with the chronic illness and incipient disability that disproportionately affect older persons. Dread diseases have to be prevented as much as possible before their onset affects functional competencies and performance.

A policy of prevention would provide a whole array of linked health services, including home care, day care, respite care, foster care, and other sheltered and protective services to address differential physical, dental, and mental health needs of older people. Available in many countries of the world, preventive health services could be paid for through a national insurance system. Institutional long-term care could be organized as a social service with an important health delivery component rather than as a health delivery system with a social service component. A well developed home-health program does not obviate the need for high quality institutional care, but rather, a range of options for patients and their families needs to be developed as part of a restructured preventive health care system. Innovative and compassionate ways of caring for the terminally ill outside the hospital or nursing home are needed such as the use of hospices and the federal channeling demonstration projects initiated in 1979. Only a well orchestrated system of physical, mental, and emotional care, which is financially underwritten by a national insurance mechanism, will be able to focus on the primary and secondary prevention of illness and disease and assure a healthier, younger age population that can meet the vicissitudes of the later years better fortified and better equipped.

The development of better environmental health conditions is another major task in promoting preventive health care for the young and old. Industrialization, mechanization, and commercialization of our country have produced hazards of grave concern to our health and well-being. Among the byproducts is pollution of our physical and social environment. An environmental health policy is a necessary part of a preventive approach to health care and adequate health care delivery policy. Such a policy to protect the aged the other community residents must include: (a) enforcement of existing air pollution codes and the establishment of new ones where needed with penalties of sufficient magnitude to discourage chronic offenders; (b) research programs to produce nonpollutant engines and other technological innovations to reduce pollution; (c) promulgation and enforcement of the highest saftey standards for the automobile industry and strict enforcement of laws aimed at the prevention of highway accidents; and (d) establishment of a national consumer code with laws to protect consumers by insuring truth in advertising, packaging, and labeling of foods and drugs.

Physical and social living. Since housing constitutes a living environment for people and provides the context for a person's daily encounters and behaviors, it takes on special meanings not only as physical shelter but also as a mark of identity. In developing social policies as mechanisms of primary prevention, seven elements can be used as criteria for determining the degree of adequacy of housing for the elderly: "age and ownership of dwelling units; the physical condition of the unit; location with regard to service; proximity to recreational, social, religious, and commercial activities; proximity to relatives and age peers; access to transportation; and safety in the neighborhood and in the dwelling" (Carp, 1976). Our housing policies should be particularly mindful of the changing needs of a new cohort of older people including: maximization of "choice"; retaining and sustaining independent living; need for personal and social services as an intrinsic part of a housing program; and need for continuing and strong federal involvement in making flexible and reasonable funding mechanisms available.

In view of the elderly's fear of crime impinging upon their living environments, it is essential that comprehensive programs of indemnification of victims of crime be established. Restitution should be made by the offender to the victim or the state, with a prohibition against recovery of damages for injuries sustained by a perpetrator. Preventive measures should include: strict enforcement of criminal laws; improved police and judicial procedures and better correctional and rehabilitation programs; orientation services and special assistance for elderly and handicapped victims or witnesses to facilitate their appearance in court; crime prevention programs aimed at increasing citizen participation and improving police training programs; expansion of law enforcement training to include segments on communicating with and understanding older persons to enable such personnel to deal effectively with the elderly.

Social/Mental Health Services as Mechanisms of Secondary and Tertiary Prevention

Just as income, health, and housing policies and programs are pillars of primary prevention for the elderly population, a critical consideration at the secondary and tertiary levels of prevention is the availability of prompt, adequate, and effective services at the point of felt need or initial crisis. What are some of the key social/ mental health services which are among the mechanisms of secondary and tertiary prevention for older persons in general and the more vulnerable elderly in particular?

Social services. There are two major federal acts that authorize the provision of social services to the elderly: the Social Security Act and the Older Americans Act. Under the Social Security Act, services for the aged (also the blind and disabled) include the following: information and referral without regard to eligibility for assistance, protective services, services to enable persons to remain in or to return to their homes or communities, supportive services that would contribute to a "satisfactory and adequate social adjustment of the individual," and services to meet health needs.

Services to the aged through the Older Americans Act include health, continuing educational, welfare, recreational, homemaker, counseling, information and referral services, transportation services where necessary to facilitate access to social services, services designed to encourage and assist older persons to use the facilities and services available to them, services designed to assist older persons in avoiding institutionalization, home health services, and any other services necessary for the general welfare of older persons.

Food programs. One program that attempts to address two problems—inadequate nutrition and social isolation—is the congregate meal. In 1972, Congress enacted the Nutrition Program for the Elderly, the purpose of which is to provide older Americans, particularly those with low incomes, low cost, nutritionally sound meals served in strategically located centers, such as schools, churches, community centers, senior citizens centers, and other public or private facilities where they can obtain other social and rehabilitative services. Besides promoting better health among the older segment of the population through improved nutrition, this program is aimed at reducing the isolation of old age, offering older Americans an opportunity to live their remaining years in dignity.

Protective services. Assistance is offered to older people who may need help in managing their money or have fears of daily living but do not yet need the elaborate legal protection of a court-appointed guardian or conservatorship. Protection for the elderly is provided in four areas: (a) protection of the life and property of the marginally functioning, non-institutionalized elderly; (b) protection of civil liberties of these same elderly; (c) protection of professional persons working in this field, to free them from burdens of anxiety about their authority and its limits; and (d) protection of the community from dangers posed by the incapacitated person (Lowy, 1979).

Geriatric day care centers and day hospitals. Day care centers are primarily social programs for frail, moderately handicapped or slightly confused older persons who need care during the day or some part of the week—either because they live alone and cannot manage altogether on their own or, by sharing some of the responsibility for their care, to relieve their family and thereby help them to keep them at home.

Group work. In use for several decades and originally performed as a spontaneous recreational activity in centers for the elderly or in golden age clubs, it has become recognized that group work demands specially trained personnel with special skills. More and more recreation centers, golden age clubs, day care centers, family agencies, general and geriatric hospitals, public welfare departments, and homes for the aged have begun to develop specialized group work services for older people who find it difficult to cope with peer and social relationships. Groups are formed with the help of a group worker and the group experience of the members is utilized for resocialization purposes. Group workers are attuned to individual needs and work with individuals in the group and also outside the group and, if necessary, make referrals to other community agencies, such as mental health clinics, where more individual treatment is available.

Group work is differentiated from group psychotherapy as it focuses on the growth and development of the "normal" healthy person, rather than on the person who suffers from emotional disorders. Group psychotherapy uses psychotherapeutic principles and techniques from individual psychotherapy as well as techniques derived from group process, while group work makes use of the group process, as it occurs, to afford each member as many growth producing experiences as possible in order to facilitate ego enhancement rather than treatment of a debilitating condition.

Suicide prevention. The highest rate of suicide occurs in white males in their 80s. The elderly, who constitute 11 percent of the population, account for 25 percent of reported suicides (5,000–8,000 yearly). This increased suicide rate in old age has been found in all Western countries. Explanations given are related to the severe loss of status that affects white men, particularly in the Western world. Butler thinks the most preventable are suicides related to depression. "Reducing the frequency of depression and providing for its effective treatment when present are the major ways of reducing suicide in old age" (Butler & Lewis, 1982).

Suicide prevention centers, many of them staffed by a small number of full-time professionals and a large number of volunteers, provide services throughout the country to potentially suicidal persons. A few such centers are located in community mental health centers. Many are operated with privately gathered funds rather than with public funding. Workers in the programs must be well acquainted with the resources of professional consultation and local community geriatric programs to which possibly suicidal older persons can be referred when indicated (Butler & Lewis, 1982).

Crisis intervention. According to crisis theory, a period of upset during crisis may be a potential turning point when the individual's vulnerability to immediate or eventual mental disorder may alter significantly. In a time of crisis there is increased openness and accessibility of the individual that can lead to both adverse and salutary consequences. The outcome of crisis intervention is dependent on a person's constitutional resilience, precrisis adjustment, coping skills engendered by others crises, general helpfulness contained within the social network, and specialized help stemming from a person's understanding of the circumstance of the crisis. Several community agencies provide crisis intervention services and crisis supports to the elderly who are often beset by physical, emotional, and social crises which result from problems of poverty, disability, illness, loss of spouse, friends, etc. Delay in responding often produces far more damaging consequences than if an immediate response had been forthcoming.

Senior centers. Providing a combination of services, contact with other elderly people, and some links with needed services, senior centers vary greatly in the kinds of programs and services offered and in the elaborateness and adequacy of physical settings. Senior centers offer programs for older people in a designated facility open three or more days a week. These programs include recreational activities, and counseling and community services (National Council on the Aging, 1979).

A senior center seeks to create a social atmosphere that acknowledges the value of human life, individually and collectively, and affirms the dignity and self-worth of the older adult. This atmosphere provides for the reaffirmation of creative potential, the power of decision making, the skills of coping and defending, and the warmth of caring, sharing, giving and supporting. The uniqueness of the senior center stems from its total concern for all older people and for the total older person. In an atmosphere of wellness, it develops strengths and encourages independence, while building interdependence and supporting unavoidable dependencies. It works with older persons not for them, enabling and facilitating their decisions and their actions, and in so doing creates and supports a sense of community which further enables older persons to continue their involvement with and contribution to the larger community.

The philosophy of the senior center movement is based on the premises that aging is a normal development process; that human beings need peers with whom they can interact and who are available as a source of encouragement and support; and that adults have the right to have a voice in determining matters in which they have a vital interest. As such, the center is a major community institution that is geared to maintaining "good" mental health and to preventing breakdown and deterioration of mental, emotional, and social functioning of older persons.

Programs to facilitate access: Information and referral. The primary purpose of specialized information and referral services is to link older people in need of help with services available in their communities. In addition, information and referral services have the potential for identifying recurrent needs and gaps in services for the elderly. For the most part, these services are provided by voluntary organizations, churches, and labor unions. Since the Older Americans Act includes a provision for federal matching funds to state approved information and referral projects, a growing number of special demonstration information and referral service projects have been funded.

Transportation. The old age transportation problem stems from four main factors: many old people cannot afford the cost of transportation; many live in areas which are poorly served by public transit; many older people have difficulty using the public transportation system; the American transportation system is based on the use of the private auto. Because they are poor, many old people live in areas which are not well served by public transportation. Because they do not have access to transit systems, they cannot go to work to supplement their incomes or make use of existing service programs either for recreational, social, or health purposes.

Participatory and action programs. These involve activities by elders to promote their well-being in work or task groups, organizations of the elderly, or in volunteer service roles under governmental or private auspices and sponsorship. In the *Foster Grandparent Program,* older people with low incomes work with children in institutions such as schools for retarded or disturbed children, infant homes, temporary care centers, and convalescent hospitals. The *Green Thumb Program* employs low income men and women in rural sections to beautify public areas such as parks and roadsides, and to help local government and community services as aides in schools and libraries.

Telephone reassurance programs. These programs provide a telephone contact for an older person who might otherwise have no outside contact for long periods of time. Recipients of this service are called at a predetermined time each day, often by older persons themselves. If the person does not answer, help is sent to the home. Usually in the event of no answer, a neighbor, relative, or nearby police or fire station is asked to make a personal check.

Lifeline. This is a formalized telephone emergency alarm system that connects older persons with a central station operator in case of emergency. The operator has lists of family, friends or back-up agencies to turn to for assistance. If older persons do not use their telephone in a 24-hour time period or reset the alarm, an emergency signal is automatically triggered to alert a central station operator (Sherwood & Morris, 1980).

Friendly visiting. Volunteers visit isolated homebound older persons on a regular schedule once, or more often, a week. They do such activities as play chess and cards, write letters, provide an arm to lean on during a shopping trip, and just sit and chat. The essential element is to provide continuing companionship for an elderly person who has no relative or friend able to do it. This kind of visiting relieves the loneliness of older people. Professional staff workers have observed that clients look better and take more interest in things outside themselves after receiving friendly visiting. Frequently, there is improvement in actual physical condition or, at least, less absorption in illness.

Peer assistance. A variation of friendly visiting, this service is particularly valuable in housing for the elderly. Neighbors check in on one another and the more physically able help those less mobile. This is often set up in a structured fashion through the manager of a housing project. Service programs are frequently included such as meals-on-wheels and organized health clinics (e.g., blood pressure checks by visiting nurses who come to the project).

Outreach. Remaining hidden from the social life and knowledge of their communities, many older people do not know of service opportunities available to them. It is necessary to seek out older people to make sure they know what services are available and where they can call for help. Outreach volunteers can be older people themselves; often they are the most effective. Some communities pay outreach workers for time and services. Sometimes outreach is provided by senior centers through the establishment of satellite neighborhood centers which can draw previously isolated older people into neighborhood activities.

Educational programs. These programs are offered on formal and informal bases in colleges and universities, adult and continuing education programs, neighborhood centers, farm and business organizations, religious organizations, museums, and civic associations. Educational programs can be divided into two types, instrumental and expressive. Instrumental programs teach skills for meeting life needs; expressive programs provide opportunities for recreation, creativity, and self-expression. Universities are increasingly paying attention to the older population and are moving not only to establish centers of gerontology but also to offer special learning programs for older students (Timmerman, 1981).

Homemaker services. Homemaker services are provided by specially trained people with skills both as homemakers and in personal care. The function of this service is to help maintain and preserve a home environment that is threatened with disruption by illness, death, social maladjustment, and other problems and to prevent premature institutionalization. Home health (aid) services refer specifically to health oriented care services and may also include some of the services performed by a homemaker. Homemaker and home health services are either hospital based (hospitals extending services into the community) or community based, with connections to other services and institutions. Services may be performed by many different kinds of private and public agencies, for example, nurse associations (voluntary, nonprofit groups delivering nursing services to the home), public health services, community agencies, and hospital based programs (U.S. House of Representatives Select Committee on Aging, 1981; White House Conference on Aging, 1982).

Social Policies and Prevention

Meeting the preventive needs of older persons in coming decades will require increasing numbers of workers at all levels who are adequately trained. Every effort must be made to support a balanced program of training of geriatric specialists in all professions, to enrich educational programs at all levels with the new knowledge that is gradually being acquired about human development and aging, to encourage public awareness of the social and economic factors that influence mental health as well as the psychological and physical aspects of aging, and to coordinate efforts to improve the quality of life of the aged now and in the future.

At present the amount and quality of training in gerontology is low among all categories of workers, both professional and paraprofessional, but especially among those personnel who spend most of their time in direct services to aged persons. While it is essential to have a core of scientific and academic personnel to train graduate students in various health and related disciplines, it is even more essential to have trainers for on-the-job training of personnel already working in institutional and community settings, most of whom are not associated with formal educational institutions. While specialized training is required, it is also important to bring an increased amount of geriatric training into the curricula of disciplines such as psychiatry, psychology, nursing, social work, and the like, for those who will not become geriatric specialists.

Training programs must also consider the need to educate the active and mobile well aged so they, in turn, can work more effectively as volunteers and/or advocates to assist the impaired aged. In addition, high school and college students who serve as volunteers in various community and institutional settings should be given training in gerontological principles. These can be especially helpful with the aged in various ethnic and non English speaking groups (National Institute of Mental Health, 1980).

Three White House Conferences on Aging (1961, 1971 and 1981) have addressed policy questions and issues and have attempted to arrive at a policy on aging. None have succeeded, though programs on a piecemeal basis have been established and enacted (for example, Medicare and the Older Americans Act). Much less have these conclaves succeeded in addressing preventive approaches to the care of the elderly. The incremental, ad hoc, curatively oriented stance is generally still prevailing, with the major exception being the social security program just recently "rescued" by congressional action.

Social policies that are preventive in orientation need to build on the institutional conception of social welfare policies, exemplified by the social insurance program. Such policies should allow for the design of health and social support programs that are predicated upon the principle of entitlement. This principle is translated into practice by tax contributions of the working population prior to any work retirement, is nationally uniform in policy but decentralized in administration and service delivery, and is free of attribution of stigma by avoiding tests of personal worthiness or financial means test.

Such social policies should postulate an array of community based health (physical and mental) and social support services that are comprehensive, continuous, and coordinated and meet the criteria of accessibility, availability, and acceptability. Accessibility means spatial arrangements that allow older persons to have access with relative ease; availability means time arrangements that allow older persons to use health and social resources when they can get to them or they can "get to older people"; acceptability means a psychological readiness to take advantage of such programs and services before a crisis occurs that could have been prevented (Lowy, 1970). Such an array of services must have several entry points in a community, yet a central coordinating mechanism (e.g., a multi-service center or an area agency on aging) must be a catalytic anchor to coordinate the multiplicity of services through case management and advocacy functions.

Despite a formidable array of programs and services for the elderly, there remain serious gaps, particularly with regard to getting comprehensive services delivered to people in an acceptable and coordinated manner. A number of questions arise. How do older people learn about what types of services exist and how they can obtain them? How accessible and acceptable are these to people? How can continuity of community care be assured in the face of fragmentation? How can services be defined in more inclusive rather than in traditional, exclusive terms? How can linkages of mental health and social services be achieved that are directly interventive, preventive, and enhancing? These are questions for which there are no easy answers now, nor in the foreseeable future, since no coordinated research strategy has as yet focused upon them.

A social policy that is preventively oriented must address the "continuum of needs" issue. Needs of people undergo changes at any time in their lives, but as people grow older their various needs tend to change more rapidly. Physiological changes intersect with social, environmental, and situational changes more frequently and coping abilities may diminish when too many losses impact the person at the same time. That is why preventive health and social policies have to plan programs and services for the comparatively well elderly. Services that provide alternatives for preventing premature breakdowns and institutionalization must be developed with built-in mechanisms for people to shift from one alternative to the other as changing needs demand.

Policies must also deal with issues of age segregation versus age integration and decide which services are better planned for people based on age criteria and which are better planned based on universal criteria (e.g., educational programs.) Prevention oriented social policies must also look at older persons as community and societal resources who can serve others (young and old) and thereby enhance their sense of being needed, wanted, and useful. By developing such a feeling many problems can be forestalled and prevented. Stress factors associated with loneliness, boredom, and feelings of uselessness can be dealt with before they become debilitating.

So far our feeble attempts at shaping social policies on aging have been curatively oriented and informed by treating the elderly as an appendage, surplus population. The demographic factors of today and even more of tomorrow will no longer permit such a shortsighted approach. Social policies of the immediate and long term future must be informed by including the elderly as part of the societal fabric. A system of preventive programs and services must be created that meets the continuously changing needs and expectations of the elderly of today and their offspring, the elderly of tomorrow.

REFERENCES

Bengtson, V.L., & Treas, J. The changing family context of mental health and aging. In J. Birren & R. Sloane (Eds.), *Handbook of mental health and aging*. Englewood Cliffs, NJ: Prentice Hall, 1980.

Brody, E.M. Women's changing roles, the aging family and long term care of older people. *National Journal*, 1979, *10*(27).

Butler, R.N., & Lewis, M.I. *Aging and mental health* (3rd ed.). St Louis: C.V. Mosby Co, 1982.

Carp, F.M. Housing and living arrangements of older people. In R. Binstock & E. Shanas (Eds.), *Handbook of aging and social sciences*. NY: Van Nostrand Reinhold, 1976.

Estes, C.L. *The aging enterprise*. San Francisco: Jossey-Bass, 1980.

Giovannoni, J.M. Prevention of child abuse and neglect: Research and policy issues. *Social Work Research and Abstracts*, 1982, *18*(3).

Kirschner, C. The aging family and crisis. *Social Casework*, 1979, (April).

Lowy, L. Models for organization of services to the aging. *Aging and Human Development*, 1970, *1*.

Lowy, L. *Challenge and promise of the later years: Social work with the aging*. NY: Harper & Row, 1979.

Lowy, L. *Social policies and programs on aging*. Lexington, MA: Lexington Books, 1980.

Lowy, L. Social group work with vulnerable older persons: A theoretical perspective. In Shura Saul (Ed.), *Group work with the frail elderly*. NY: Haworth Press, 1983.

Miller, D.A. The sandwich generation: Adult children of the aging. *Social Work*, 1981.

National Council on the Aging. *Standards for senior centers*. Washington, DC: National Council on the Aging, 1979.

National Institute of Mental Health. *A preliminary report on the development and implementation of a federal manpower policy for the field of aging*. Washington, DC: U.S. Government Printing Office, 1980.

Timmerman, S. *Education for older persons in the U.S.A.* Paper presented at the International Conference of Gerontology, Hamburg, West Germany, 1981.

Sherwood, S., & Morris, J.N. *Effects of an emergency alarm and response system for the aged* (Final report, Part 1). Boston: Hebrew Rehabilitation Center for the Aged, 1980.

U.S. House of Representatives Select Committee on Aging. *White house conference on aging, 1981 technical committee report*. Washington, DC: U.S. Government Printing Office, 1981.

White House Conference on Aging. *Final report of the 1981 white house conference on aging*. Washington, DC: U.S. Department of Health and Human Services, 1982.

The Status of Preventive
Care for the Aged: A Meta-Analysis

Laura B. Wilson
Sharon Simson
Kim McCaughey

ABSTRACT. One response to the growing needs of the elderly is to expand the scope of preventive care from the younger and middle aged cohorts to include an emphasis on preventive care for older people. In the past it has been difficult to consider prevention and aging as concepts which could co-exist because we can neither cure nor prevent aging. The potential of preventive care to improve, maintain, or lessen decline in the quality of life of the elderly has not been included in the definition or mainstream of prevention activities. This study identifies and reviews research and programmatic activities which have been reported in the literature over the last ten years in the area of prevention and aging. Topical areas and methodological approaches are explored to define what has been considered appropriate preventive care for the elderly. An evaluation process, meta-analysis, is used to assess the therapeutic effect and overall effectiveness of techniques in prevention and aging. These findings can be used in formulating future initiatives related to aging and prevention.

In the past twenty years, the delivery of health and social services to the elderly population has been profoundly impacted upon by a number of factors. Technological advances in science, medicine, nutrition and related areas have increased the ability to prolong life (U.S. Senate, 1982). This increase in life span has been accom-

Laura B. Wilson is Assistant Professor and Director, Gerontology Services Administration, University of Texas Health Science Center, Dallas. Kim McCaughey is at the University of Texas Health Science Center, Dallas. Sharon Simson is Assistant Professor of Mental Health Service at Hahnemann University, Philadelphia.

Requests for reprints may be sent to the senior author, Laura B. Wilson, University of Texas Health Science Center, 5323 Harry Hines Boulevard, Dallas, TX 75235.

23

panied by a host of problems for the elderly which include their vulnerability to multiple chronic illnesses and susceptability to environmental hazards, the inability of the culture to provide additional social roles and responsibilities, and the inadequacy of health and social services to meet emerging needs (Brody, 1979). All of these problems and issues are compounded further by population growth patterns which indicate a growing percentage of elderly in our population who live increasingly longer and make multiple demands upon the service system (Allan & Brotman, 1981).

One feasible response to these changes and growing needs of the elderly is to expand the scope of preventive care from the younger and middle aged cohorts to include an emphasis on preventive care for older people. Preventive approaches have been designed and used effectively with younger populations in a number of ways including eliminating the underlying cause of a disease or disability, providing for early detection, encouraging prompt treatment in order to avoid disability, and providing for rehabilitation (Doll, 1978). Despite the fact that these approaches could be applied to an older age cohort, preventive care has often been seen as the purview of younger populations only. Historically, health and social services have been directed toward meeting acute care needs and effecting a cure as result of the intervention. Preventive approaches were tied to this process and meant to reduce the incidence of acute care needs in the population through actions focusing on health maintenance and improvement. As these approaches do not have as a primary target the noncurative, long term care needs associated with the chronic disease processes of the elderly (German, 1981), this population was not seen as appropriate to receive many preventive services. They could not be completely cured or rehabilitated. In addition, many preventive techniques must commence early in life to have an overall effect on the later years. This combination of factors has limited programs and research in prevention and aging. The potential of preventive care to improve, maintain, or lessen decline in the quality of life of the elderly has not been included in the definition or mainstream of prevention activities.

The purpose of this study is to provide an overview of the current state of the art which can serve as a foundation for determining future initiatives which focus on prevention and the elderly. This study identifies and reviews research and programmatic activities which have been reported in the literature over the last ten years in the area of prevention and aging. Topical areas and methodological approaches are explored to define what has been considered appropriate preventive care for the elderly. In addition, an evaluation process, meta-analysis, is used to assess the therapeutic effect and overall effectiveness of techniques in prevention and aging. These findings can be used by clinicians, researchers, educators, administrators, and older persons to assist them in formulating future initiatives related to aging and prevention.

LITERATURE REVIEW

During the last ten years studies have tended to present singular program efforts or individual concepts regarding prevention for the aged. They have often used a descriptive approach and few have built upon existing literature or provided an empirical review of previous work. Among the specific topical areas explored are: action for prolonging life (Robbins, 1980), early assessment (Taylor, 1980), screening (Morrison, 1980), preventing falls and accidents (Morris, 1980), reducing cardiovascular risk (Kannel, 1978), preventing confusion (Remakus, 1981), reducing brain dysfunction (Livesley, 1978), oral dentistry rehabilitation (Langer, 1978), health education (Dinsmore, 1979), and nutrition (Seeman, 1981). In order to acquaint readers with some of the past work done on aging and prevention, five types of interventions from the aging and prevention literature are reviewed.

Nursing Interventions

Nurses are one group which has been active in defining prevention related to the elderly. Combs (1978) discusses preventive care for the elderly as a means for minimizing the effects of existing problems and preventing further problems. From her nursing perspective she suggests several areas of importance in prevention for the elderly which include health habits, nutrition and safety. Griffin (1980) also presents a nursing view and discusses primary and holistic health care related to the aged. Wellness is emphasized rather than illness. Linn (1979) discusses key preventive measures for the elderly in maintaining independence of life style. The importance of the nurse's role in health education, investigation of home environments, and counseling regarding problems of daily living are emphasized.

Physician Interventions

Physicians have also taken a role in beginning to define prevention related to the elderly. Shukla (1981) indicates that a team approach is needed to review physical, psychological, and social problems of the elderly. Named as leader of this team is the general medical practitioner. He identifies some of the preventive measures needed for the elderly to include reassessment of prescribing habits, good communication, patient and family education, control of hypertension, and information and referral services. Allen (1979), a general practitioner, asserts that the best approach to healthier lives for the aged is primary prevention rather than secondary, crisis intervention. He also suggests that life style changes alone may effect some health improvements for the aged. Breslow (1977) provides a lifelong cost-effective and health-effective program which identifies health goals and professional services throughout the life span. Robbins (1980) makes a distinction between prolonging life until a disease develops and preventing conditions which contribute to premature mortality. He identifies smoking, drinking, obesity, activity, homicide, suicide, accidents, and firearm control as areas of patient education which will help to improve the quality of life. He also emphasizes that the physician's role is only one part of a prevention plan and that the culture as a whole must grapple with these issues.

Mental Health Interventions

A large portion of the literature in prevention for the elderly focuses on mental health. The chronically ill, institutionalized, and isolated elderly are particularly vulnerable to depression, suicidal thoughts, and confusion. Eisenberg (1981) provides a research framework for evaluating the promotion of mental health and the prevention of mental illness. One area in which he strongly recommends intervention is that of social networking. He found that both psychological and physical symptoms could be reduced by strong social bonding. Bayne (1978) discusses prevention and management of confusion in the elderly. He emphasizes understanding of home conditions as a means of preventing future emergencies. Coetzee (1980) outlines a program of prevention related to depressive illness among the elderly. The program utilizes community referrals to identify possible depression cases among the elderly.

Community Services and Program Interventions

Closely related to mental health interventions are community-based prevention services and programs. These services are primarily psychosocial in nature and are operated by members of the social work and psychology professions. For example, Blackwell (1980) describes services which focus on teaching the elderly to cope with the aging process. Abrahams (1979) discusses age-integrated psychosocial rehabilitation in long term geriatric patients. Patients hospitalized for long term illness are given remotivating therapy which impacts on their overall health and prevents further problems, thus improving their quality of life. One social service intervention discussed by Beck (1982) was manipulation of the environment in the form of therapeutic cognitive activity. In this set of activities, the nursing home setting was the environment and residents were encouraged to be in greater control. Schaie (1981) takes the approach that many of the social and mental health difficulties of the aged are the result of stereotypes which become self-fulfilling prophecies. He suggests providing training and education to dispel such myths both for the older population and for the health and social service personnel working with them.

Future Interventions

A number of articles have appeared in the literature which focus on future perspectives related to aging and prevention. Sir Richard Doll (1978) points to changes in smoking and eating habits as preventive measures which have vastly affected the incidence of lung cancer and myocardial infarction in the aged. He acknowledges that although preventive efforts over the last several decades have been effective, new environmental occupational hazards have lead to additional and increasing prevention problems. Wynder (1977) details the effects that having a healthy older population can have on society. These effects include reduced medical care, more health care personnel spending time on prevention, conversion of acute care facilities to meet housing needs, and government savings converted into social benefits. In short, a healthy older population would be less of a burden and more productive members of society.

While this literature provides some insight into specific preventive interventions and viewpoints, it does not permit comparisons of methods or analyze the overall state of the art in prevention and aging. The next section describes a process for achieving this assessment.

METHOD

In order to assess the status of preventive care activities, an evaluation of the prevention literature was conducted. A literature search was completed using MEDLARS (Medical Literature Analysis and Retrieval System) for the period from August, 1972 to August, 1982. Medlars is a data base maintained by the National Library of Medicine and contains references to bibliographic citations from over 3000 biomedical journals in the United States and 70 foreign countries. Key words used in the search were "prevention" cross-referenced with "aging," "elderly," "self-help," "self-care," "geriatrics," and "primary care."

A pool of 108 articles was retrieved through this system and reviewed for method, outcome measures and modality. All studies were summarized and recorded. From this group 32 studies evidencing a research design were identified. From this group, 13 controlled experimental and quasi experimental studies were selected for meta-analysis (Campbell & Stanley, 1963). Selection criteria included (1) the use of an experimental design; (2) a study population 55 years or older; (3) and the use of an independent variable as a prevention protocol with dependent variable compliance, progress, or change in health or social status of the older client or patient. In summary, each study was required to test, through an empirical method, the effects of prevention techniques on the aged.

The 13 studies selected were evaluated through meta-analysis. According to Glass (1977, p. 21), meta-analysis is "the attitude of data analysis applied to quantitative summaries of individual experiments." Meta-analysis is a "perspective that uses many techniques of measurement and statistical analysis"; it is "the statistical analysis of the summary of findings of many empirical studies" (Glass, 1977, p. 21). Meta-analysis is quantitative, does not prejudge research findings in terms of research quality, and seeks general conclusions. Meta-analysis looks at the overall effectiveness of previously completed research in a given area by calculating the effect size (ES) for each dependent variable (i.e., compliance, progress, change) identified. This process permits the comparison of research which varies in design, format, and population size. Meta-analysis provides a means of integrating multiple findings to make decisions about the overall benefits of prevention approaches for the aged.

Effect size (Glass, 1977) is the difference between the mean of the experimental group $(\overline{X}_e)$ and the mean of the control group $(\overline{X}_c)$ divided by the standard deviation of the control group (S_c). The basic equation is:

$$\text{Effect size} = \frac{(\overline{X}_e - \overline{X}_c)}{S_c}.$$

The difference between the means is converted to a Z-score which describes the status of the experimental versus the control group. The calculated effect size can then be converted to a percentile rank using the standard normal table. Thus, a number of diverse reports on prevention can be compared to assess effectiveness and improvement. This approach was used to test significance for each dependent variable. The mean ES was calculated and tested against the null hypothesis of no difference (ES = 0).

RESULTS

The initial literature search provided 108 articles on prevention and aging. From this group, 32 studies were identified as having a research design. These studies are summarized in Table 1 which records design, study population, sample size, preventive modality, objectives, outcome measures and findings. Review of the 32 designs showed four categories of methodological approach which included: survey questionnaire (6 studies), experimental or quasi-experimental (13 studies), program evaluation (11 studies), and preexisting data bank analysis (2 studies).

Of these 32 studies, 13 were classified as control or experimental designs which were appropriate for meta-analysis. These studies were in the following prevention areas: exercise, two; psychosocial, seven; crime, one; nutrition, one; cable tv patient education, one; and dentistry, one. Of the 13 experimental designs, enough data was provided in 8 studies to permit meta-analysis.

All eight of the studies investigated favored the experimental group in effect size calculation. Effect size (ES) is calculated in Table 2. It contains a list of studies and indicates prevention measures and the size of the experimental and control groups. Within categories of prevention the limited number of acceptable cases necessitated dividing the studies into two categories which would assess psychosocial interventions as compared to health related in-

Table I: Summary of Prevention and Aging Literature with Research Designs

Study	Prevention Modality	Sample	Objectives	Design	Outcome	Findings
Abrahams et al., 1979	Age-integrated psychosocial rehabilitation	Random; 12 long term care patients of VA hospital	Study effects of psychosocial rehabilitation on behavioral functioning of aged	Sickness Impact Profile Population Evaluation, pre, post test	Dysfunction score	Increased social interaction, increased mobility
Allen, 1979	Preventive care in general practice	Random; 56 patients	Motivation techniques to change health patterns	Pretest posttest health habit questionnaire survey	Motivational rating	High rate of discontinuation of poor health habits
hAloia, 1981	Prevention of bone loss through exercise	Random; 62 subjects	Reduction in skeletal problems in aging	Prospective experimental vs. control; pre, post, & follow-up	Photon absorptiometry	Increase in body calcium
hAniansson et al., 1980	Physical training influences on muscle strength	Random; 12, 70 year old men	Test exercise as a means of influencing muscle strength	Experimental vs. control; pre, post & follow-up	Muscle strength, aerobic capacity	Increased aerobic capacity & increased muscle strength
Bilderbeck et al., 1981	Food habit change	Non-Random; over 60 100 subjects	Define alterations in food habits	Posttest	Dietary change	Changes made to improve health or for convenience
Blackwell & Hunt, 1980	Mental health prevention	Non-Random; 223	Promote mental habits through positive view of aging	Posttest	Attitude	Improved sense of self
Brockbank & Broukova, 1980	Screening	Random; 43 patients	Assess multiple screening procedures	Screening evaluation	Disease identification	Detection of abnormality

h = Health study used in final analysis

Table 1 (Continued)

Study	Prevention Modality	Sample	Objectives	Design	Outcome	Findings
Coetzee, 1980	Case finding	Random; 300	To effect casefinding and secondary prevention of depression	Data bank mortality analysis	Reduction in death rate	Need aggressive preventive measures
de Vries, 1979	Exercise	Random; 200, 58-88 years	Medical screening and assessment of tolerance	Exercise testing evaluation	Target heart rate blood pressure	Improved vital capacity
Dinsmore, 1979	Health education	Non-Random; 150	Medical maintenance & promotion	Evaluation questionnaire post test	Improved knowledge	Maintained activity level
PEvans & Jaurequy, 1982	Phone therapy	Random; 84	Provide therapy for social & personal problems of the aged	Experimental vs. control	Personal Assessment of Roles, Wakefield Depression Scale	Improved task centered goal attainment
Fitton, 1980	Health visiting	Convenience Sample; 71	Evaluate health visitors concept of visit	Survey questionnaire	Preconceived plan	Health visitors have structured concept of visit
Futrell & Jones, 1977	Health manpower attitudes	Random; 157	Assess attitudes toward elderly	Survey questionnaire	Test knowledge	Health professionals have some positiveness in attitude
German, 1981	Health care instructions	Random; 350	Assess influence of approaches to care instructions	Household survey questionnaire	Compliance	Effective health education strategies suggested
Hale, 1981	Hypertension screening	Random; 4247	Screening to reduce morbidity	Longitudinal screening & follow-up evaluation	Reduced blood pressure	Effective control of blood pressure

p = Psycho-social study used in final analysis

Table 1 (Continued)

Study	Prevention Modality	Sample	Objectives	Design	Outcome	Findings
PJohnson, 1981	Reality orientation	Non-Random; 98	Improved orientation of elderly	Experimental vs. control; pre & posttest	Test score for reality orientation	High improvement
Kannel & Gordon, 1978	Risk factor prediction	Random; 5209	Prevention of cardiovascular disease	Exploratory, follow-up evaluation	Mortality rate	Decreased risk
PLanger & Rodin, 1979	Memory training	Random; 45 nursing home residents	Memory improvement through reward	Experimental vs. control; pre, post & follow-up	Lag test scores of memory	Improved memory & social adjustment
PLanger & Rodin, 1976	Therapeutic effects of cognitive activity	Random; 91, 65-90 years	Increase patient control over environment to improve health	Experimental vs. control; pre, post & follow-up	Self report of sense of control, nurse rating of activity	Self care group were more satisfied
Leeder et al., 1981	Assessment	Random; 259	Identification of remediable confusion	Experimental vs. control Ladder	Number of cases perception	Reversed confusion
Leviton & Santa Maria, 1979	Adult health training	Random; 34	Improved health knowledge & activity	Evaluation survey / Cantril Ladder	Change in self perception	Improved well being
Miller & Le Lieuvre, 1982	Reduction of chronic pain	Non-Random; 7	Use attention & praise to increase exercise	Exercise quota pre, post evaluation	McGill-Melzack Inventory Scale	Lower pain behavior but no increase in activity
Morris & Issacs,	Fall prevention	Random; 236	Identify fall prevention methods	Descriptive statistics/ data bank analysis	Lower falls	Promotion of safety

p = Psycho-social study used in final analysis

Table 1 (Continued)

Study	Prevention Modality	Sample	Objectives	Design	Outcome	Findings
Norton & Courlander, 1982	Crime prevention	Random; 152	Examine effect of police patrol & crime education on fear of crime	Experimental vs. control	Crime belief	Lower fear for patrol but higher for education program
Rae & Burke, 1978	Nutrition counseling	Random; 92	Effect of community nutrition service	Experimental vs. control	Nutrition status	Increased awareness
Reifler et al., 1981	Evaluation program	Random; 76	Revealing undetected illness for cognitive impaired	Descriptive	Self reported improvement, cognitive test	Cognitive & motor improvement
pSalzer, 1977	Cable tv education	Random; 195	Determine if televised health messages could effective stimulate behavorial response	Experimental vs. control modular demonstrations	Health seeking behavior	Increased use of preventive measures
Salber et al.,	Dental prevention	Random; 1685	Increase preventive behaviors	Panel, household survey, experimental vs. control	Number of visits	Increase in preventive actions
Stuart & Mackey,	Mobile service screening	Random; 616	Enhance health status through education & screening	Screening evaluation	Number served	Increased use of services
Stoller, 1982	Support systems	Random; 753 nonstitutionalized aged	Examine sources of potential help persons 65+	Interview survey questionnaire	Comprehensive Assessment Referral & Evaluation Score	Coping strategies are limited
Wallach et al., 1979	Intergenerational rehabilitation	Random; 175 patients 235 students	Develop means to lessen isolation & increase social interaction	Pretest posttest evaluation	Sickness Impact Profile Score	Increased social interaction, mobility
pZarit et al., 1981	Memory training	Random; 42	Improve memory of elderly	Experimental vs. control; pre, posttest	Recall	Improved recall

h = Health study used in final analysis
p = Psycho-social study used in final analysis

Table II

The Effects of Preventive Intervention
for the Aged

Study	Nature of Experimental Group Intervention	Size of Experimental (n_1) and Control Group (n_2)	Outcome Effect Size[a]
Aloia, 1981	Photon absorptiometry tests on nursing home subjects, 36 months	n_1 = 12 n_2 = 17	.50
Aniansson et al., 1980	Physical training for 45 minutes, 3 times a week for 12 weeks. Static & dynamic exercise	n_1 = 12 n_2 = 12	.33
Langer & Rodin, 1976	Increase nursing home resident control over environment through care routine	n_1 = 47 n_2 = 44	.12
Langer & Rodin, 1979	Reward tokens given in testing process to enhance recall	n_1 = 30 n_2 = 15	.64
Evans & Jaurequy, 1982	Phone counseling to alleviate depression for the blind	n_1 = 42 n_2 = 42	.95
Johnson et al., 1981	Classroom reality orientation sessions	n_1 = 75 n_2 = 23	.05
Salzer et. al., 1977	Cable tv used to inform about prevention services	n_1 = 120 n_2 = 75	.77
Zarit et al., 1981	Groups taught memory training strategies	n_1 = 21 n_2 = 21	.30

[a]All of the outcome effect sizes favor the experimental group.

terventions. The six psychosocial interventions tested hypotheses concerning memory, counseling, and reality orientation. The mean change in psychosocial outcome was .41 ($p < .01$). The two health related studies had a mean outcome change of .53 ($p < .01$). Across the 8 estimates of ES, the mean change in psychosocial interventions vs. health status interventions is .45 ($p < 01$). These figures represent a highly positive response to preventive interventions. The experimental groups which had interventions applied to them were more successful than control groups by almost one-half standard deviation. These findings are consistent across the studies.

DISCUSSION

Professionals seeking to assess the value of prevention activities related to the elderly should review these findings with care. Clearly, both psychosocial and health related interventions had a positive effect on the elderly. However, a final outcome showing only positive results for the experimental group gives rise to questions. The possible effect on the ES of unpublished prevention study results, if they were available, must be considered. Presumably, the majority of negative prevention studies do not reach publication and therefore, their effect on the outcome measure is not experienced. Smith (1980) assessed this issue by reviewing unpublished theses versus published meta-analysis literature. He discovered that the ES calculated in published research was one-third larger than that of unpublished studies. These factors must be taken into consideration when reviewing effect size and assessing its value for service planning.

While the overall results of both the psychosocial interventions and health interventions are positive, the issue of the variation in tested populations and the importance of individual circumstances must be considered. The interventions described usually were performed either on institutionalized or non-institutionalized populations, not both. These populations must be considered independently because of their differing capabilities to respond to intervention activities. The ability to control the environment changes in these two groups. In addition, the overall age and disease patterns of the tested populations varies considerably and will influence outcomes.

Individual personalities and life styles of the aged must also be considered independent of the meta-analysis findings. The economic status of the aged person, the availability of informal and formal support networks, the degree and multiplicity of chronic illness, and the degree of psychological impairment will impact greatly on the success of any prevention technique. These factors must be taken into consideration before needlessly undertaking a prevention approach which impedes the current life style and coping strategies of an older person and his or her family.

This review and meta-analysis of the available literature indicates that there is still a long way to go in the field of prevention and aging. The number of studies is limited and those representing true experimental designs from which conclusions can be drawn is even smaller. Given the high potential in the elderly for multiple psychosocial and physical problems as well as the current advances in understanding of the psychological and physical processes in aging, more prevention approaches should be in evidence and tested. The capability to assess preventive methods and to determine the most successful approaches takes on growing importance and becomes increasingly dependent on the availability of good research data. Such research data will provide a foundation for expanding the definition of preventive care to include the elderly as an important target population.

REFERENCES

Abrahams, J. P., Wallach, H., & Direns, S. Behavioral improvement in long-term geriatric patients during an age-integrated psychosocial rehabilitation program. *Journal of American Geriatrics Society,* 1979, *27*(5), 218-220.

Allan, C., & Brotman, H. *Chartbook on aging in America.* The 1981 White House Conference on Aging. Washington, D. C.: The 1981 White House Conference on Aging, 1981.

Allen, D. W. Preventive care in general practice. *Australian Family Physician,* 1979, *8,* 118-133.

Aloia, J. F. Exercise and skeletal health. *Journal of the American Geriatrics Society,* 1981, *29*(3), 104-106.

Aniansson, A. Physical training in old men. *Age and Aging,* 1980, *9,* 186-187.

Bayne, J. R. D. Management of confusion in elderly persons. *Canadian Medical Association Journal,* 1978, *118,* 139-141.

Beck, P. Two successful interventions in nursing homes: The therapeutic effects of cognitive activity. *The Gerontologist,* 1982, *22*(4), 378-383.

Bilderbeck, M., Holdsworth, M., Purves, R., & Davies, L. Changing food habits among 100 elderly men and women in the United Kingdom. *Journal of Human Nutrition,* 1981, *35,* 448-455.

Blackwell, D. L., & Hunt, S. S. Mental health services reaching out to older persons. *Journal of Gerontological Social Work,* 1980, *2*(4), 281-288.

Breslow, L., & Somers, A. R. The lifetime health-monitoring program. *The New England Journal of Medicine,* 1977, *296*(11), 601-608.

Brockbank, K., & Brouckova, V. Multiple screening for somatic disease among long-term psychogeriatric patients. *The British Journal of Clinical Practice,* 1977, *3,* 7-13.

Brody, E. M. Long term care for the aged: Promises and prospects. *Health and Social Work,* 1979, *4*(1).

Campbell, D. T., & Stanley, J. C. *Experimental and quasi-experimental designs for research.* Chicago: Rand McNally, 1963.

Coetzee, D. Secondary prevention of depressive illness among the elderly. *SA Mediese Tydskrif,* 1980, October 4, 571-574.

Combs, K. L. Preventive care in the elderly. *American Journal of Nursing,* 1978, *78,* 1339-1341.

Craig, T. J., & Lin, S. P. Mortality among elderly psychiatric patients: Basis for preventive intervention. *Journal of the American Geriatrics Society,* 1981, *29*(4), 181-185.

de Vries, H. A. Tips on prescribing exercise regimens for your older patient. *Geriatrics,* 1979, *34*(4), 77-81.

Dinsmore, P. A. A health education program for elderly residents in the community. *Nursing Clinics of North America,* 1979, *14*(4), 585-593.

Doll, R. Prevention: Some future perspectives. *Preventive Medicine,* 1978, *7,* 486-497.

Eisenberg, L. A research framework for evaluating the promotion of mental health and prevention of mental illness. *Public Health Reports,* 1981, *96*(13), 3-19.

Evans, R., & Jaurequy, B. Phone therapy outreach for blind elderly *The Gerontologist*, 1982, *22*(1), 32-35.

Fitton, J. Health visiting the aged. *Health Visitor*, 1980 *53*, 524-525.

German, P. S. Delivery of care to older people: Issues and outlooks. *Topics in Clinical Nursing*, 1981, *3*(1), 1-13.

Glass, G. V. Integrating findings: The meta-analysis of research. In L. S. Schulman (Ed.), *Review of research in education* (Vol. 5). Itasca, Ill: F. E. Peacock, 1977.

Griffin, M. M. Holistic approach to the health care of an elderly client. *Journal of Gerontological Nursing*, 1980, *6*(4), 193-196.

Hale, W. E., Marks, R. G., & Stewart, R. B. Screening for hypertension in an elderly population: The Framingham study. *Bulletin of the New York Academy of Medicine*, 1978, *54*(6), 573-591.

Johnson, C. H. The comparative effectiveness of three versions of classroom reality orientation. *Age and Aging*, 1981, *10*, 33-35.

Kannel, W. B., & Gordon, T. Evaluation of cardiovascular risk in the elderly: The Framingham study. *Bulletin of the New York Academy of Medicine*, 1978, *54*(6), 573-591.

Langer, A. Long-term preventive aspects in oral rehabilitation of adults and elderly: Part 1. *Journal of Oral Rehabilitation*, 1978, *5*, 129-138.

Langer, E., & Rodin, J. The effects of choice and enhanced personal responsibility: A field experiment in an institutional setting. *Journal of Personality and Social Psychology*, 1976, *34*, 191-198.

Langer, E., Rodin, J., Beck, P., Weinman, C., & Spitzer, L. Environmental determinants of memory improvement in late adulthood. *Journal of Personality and Social Psychology*, 1979, *37*, 2003-2013.

Leeder, S. R., Gunasekera, D., & Gibson, R. M. Preventing acute confusional states in elderly patients. *Australian Family Physician*, 1981, *10*, 129-130.

Leviton, D., & Santa Maria, L. The adults health and developmental program: Descriptive and evaluative data. *The Gerontologist*, 1979, *19*(6), 534-543.

Linn, J. T. Practicing prevention for the elderly. *Australian Family Physician*, 1980, *8*, 305-313.

Livesley, B. The treatment and prevention of brain failure. *Age and Aging*, 1978, Supplement, 27-30.

Miller, C., & Le Lieuvre, R. A method to reduce chronic pain in elderly nursing home residents. *The Gerontologist*, 1982, *22*(3), 314-317.

Morris, E. V., & Issacs, B. The prevention of falls in a geriatric hospital. *Age and Aging*, 1980, *9*, 181-185.

Morrison, J. D. Geriatric preventive health maintenance. *Journal of the American Geriatrics Society*, 1980, *28*(3), 314-317.

Norton, L., & Courlander, M. Fear of crime among the elderly: The role of crime prevention. *The Gerontologist*, 1982, *22*(4), 388-393.

Rae, J., & Burke, A. L. Counseling the elderly on nutrition in a community health care system. *Journal of the American Geriatrics Society*, 1978, *8*(3), 130-135.

Reifler, B., Larson, E., Cox G., & Featherstone, H. Treatment results at a multi-specialty clinic for the impaired elderly and their families. *Journal of the American Geriatrics Society*, 1978, *8*(3), 130-135.

Remakus, B., & Shelly, R. How to prevent confusion in hospitalized elderly. *Geriatrics*, 1981, *36*(6), 121-123.

Robbins, J. A. Preaching in your practice: What to tell patients to help them live longer. *Primary Care*, 1980, *7*(4), 549-562.

Salber, E., Brogan, L., Greene, S. B., & Feldman, J. J. Utilization of services for preventable disease: A case study of dental care in a southern rural area of the United States. *International Journal of Epidemiology*, 1978, *7*(2), 163-173.

Salber, E. The use of cable television as a tool in health educators of the elderly screening. *Health Education Monographs*, 1977, *5*(4), 363-378.

Schaie, K. W. Psychological changes from midlife to early old age: Implications for the maintenance of mental health. *American Journal of Orthopsychiatry*, 1981, *51*(2), 199-218.

Seeman, E., & Briggs, B. L. Dietary prevention of bone loss in the elderly. *Geriatrics*, 1981, *36*(9), 71-79.

Shukla, R. B. The role of the primary care team in the care of the elderly. *The Practitioner*, 1981, *225*, 791-797.

Smith, M. L. Publication bias and meta-analysis. *Evaluation in Education*, 1980, *4*, 22-24.

Stoller, E. P. Sources of support for the elderly during illness. *Health and Social Work*, 1982, *7*(2), 111-121.

Stuart, M., & Mackey, K. J. Mobile center links providers with isolated senior citizens. *Hospitals*, 1978, *52*, 101-105.

Taylor, V. E. Decubitus prevention through early assessment. *Journal of Gerontological Nursing*, 1980, *6*(7), 389-391.

U. S. Senate, Special Committee on Aging. *Developments in Aging: 1981*. Washington, D. C.: U. S. Government Printing Office, 1982.

Wallach, H. F., Kelley, F., & Abrahams, J. P. Psychosocial rehabilitation for chronic geriatric patients: An intergenerational approach. *The Gerontologist*, 1979, *19*(5), 464-470.

Wynder, E., & Kristein, M. M. Suppose we died young, late in life. . . ? *Journal of the American Medical Association*, 1977, *238*(14), 1507.

Zarit, S. H., Cole, K. D., & Guider, B. L. Memory training strategies and subjective complaints of memory in the aged. *The Gerontologist*, 1981, *21*(2), 158-164.

Healthy Aging through Knowledge
and Self-Care

Evelynn C. Gioiella

ABSTRACT. The normal aging process results in physical and psychosocial changes which can compromise health. Knowledge of these changes and self-care activities which limit their impact on health status are essential for prevention in the elderly. To stimulate and support these self-care behaviors teaching, counseling, screening, referral, and activity oriented human services are needed.

The 1980 Census reported 25,544,133 people over 65 years of age in the United States population. This is a 28 percent increase in ten years and represents 11.3 percent of the total population. Life expectancy has also risen. The average 65 year old male can now expect to live to 78 and the female to 82. The longer life expectancy in women has resulted in three women to every two men over the age of 65. The gain in life expectancy means that there are now millions of "young-old" in their sixties and seventies who with appropriate services focused on prevention of disability can lead vigorous, satisfying lives. Recent studies indicate that 95 percent of the over 65 age group live at home (Siegel, 1976). Only 14 percent of the population living at home is restricted in mobility enough to be considered homebound (Shanas, 1980).

Aging is a lifelong process. Understanding of this process in the later years of life is still largely theoretical. Separating the effects of normal age changes and disease in late life is difficult. Research has found some changes in human structure and function to be universal to aging. Individuals manifest these changes in different degrees. Diversity is the hallmark of the elderly; however, some degree of

Evelynn C. Gioiella is Dean and Professor of Nursing, City College of New York School Nursing, New York City.

Reprints may be requested from Evelynn C. Gioiella, School of Nursing, City College of New York, Convent Avenue at 138th Street, New York, NY 10031.

change due to the aging process occurs in everyone. Maintaining health in the face of these changes is the aim of prevention.

Prevention of illness and disability involves activities that support positive health behaviors. These behaviors can be encouraged, initiated and taught by health care givers; however, regular practice of these behaviors depends on the elderly being concerned with their own health status. Activities undertaken by care givers, therefore, should focus on self-care and the maintenance of maximum independence. Older people themselves must develop an understanding of the aging process and health promoting activities as a basis for self-care.

This paper summarizes briefly the physical and psychosocial changes that result from the normal aging process. Self-care activities which the older person can perform to maintain health while experiencing these changes are presented. Services that care-givers can provide to promote and support self-care are also described.

CHANGES RELATED TO NORMAL AGING AND HEALTH MAINTENANCE BEHAVIORS

Physical Changes

Cells decrease in number with age. Cell loss occurs in most organs and tissues including muscle, brain, lungs, spleen, kidney and liver. Cell structure also changes. Non-dividing cells in the nervous system, heart, musculoskeletal system and other organs repair or replace damaged intercellular elements on a regular basis. With aging, this ability to repair and replace is decreased. Defects accumulate and functioning is compromised. Mitotic or dividing cells also change with age. These cells show an increase in the time it takes to divide and a buildup of cellular debris which leads to gradual degeneration.

With increased age there is an overall increase in body fat. Subcutaneous fat is lost; however, fat in and around the viscera is increased. Lean body mass (muscle tissue and nerves) decreases as the aging process progresses. This reduces metabolizing tissue, resulting in a loss of basal heat production. Body weight reflects the changes in body tissue composition. Men show a steady decline in weight after age 55. Women show an increase until age 60, then a plateau, followed by gradual decline. Connective tissues collagen and elastin change with age. They become more dense and less elastic, less able to respond to stress and the need for flexibility. Decreased pulmonary compliance and decreased vascular elasticity are two examples of the resulting changes.

Loss of bone mass is another characteristic of the aging process. Bone growth continues well into the sixth decade producing greater bone thickness throughout the skeleton. However, despite bone growth, reabsorption of the interior of long and flat bones occurs at a faster rate. This loss of bone mass (osteoporosis) occurs more in females than males and may be influenced by estrogen, calcium, and exercise.

Cartilage layers which protect joints erode over time. Bone may come into contact with bone causing damage, pain and eventual fibrosis. Irregular growth of the margins of joints may occur. Synovial fluid becomes more viscous. Intervertebral discs lose water contributing to loss of height. Osteoarthritic changes occur throughout the vertebral column.

Wrinkling of skin is a hallmark of the aging process. Several factors are involved including changes in elasticity, loss of subcutaneous fat, repeated use of underlying muscles and nutritional status.

Sebaceous glands decrease their level of functioning with age, especially in women after menopause. This may be related to reduced gonadal and adrenal androgen production. Changes in sweat glands also contribute to dryer skin.

Sensory nerves to the skin are reduced in number with age. Wound healing is retarded. Nail growth declines. Hair loss accompanies aging due to loss of circulation to the scalp. In men hereditary baldness may also occur. Axillary and pubic hair is lost. Leg and arm hair may also decrease. Remaining hair may become grey, thin and fine. Some very old people may be virtually hairless.

Changes in the cardiovascular system include lipofusion build-up in cardiac cells. Muscle as a percentage of heart tissue decreases. In the ventricle, fibrosis and sclerosis occur. Fat infiltration also develops. Less efficient functioning is the result.

Resting heart rate remains unchanged. Heart rate increase related to stress is less effective with age and return to normal takes longer. Increased irritability of the myocardium may produce extra systoles and various arrhythmias. Cardiac output decreases slightly and circulation time increases. Work capacity measured by oxygen consumption gradually decreases.

The vascular system exhibits progressive changes with age.

Thickening and fibrosis of large arteries occurs. Cross linkages develop, trapping lipids and other materials. Vessel dilation, rigidity and tortuosity develop due to changes in collagen and elastin. Systolic blood pressure increases with age. Diastolic blood pressure also increases but at a much slower rate. A widening of pulse pressure results. Following exercise and changes in position, return to normal blood pressure is slowed.

Normal immune function declines with age. The exact nature and mechanism of this decline is not yet understood.

Many changes occur in the oral cavity. Teeth suffer from attrition and gradually change in composition.

Taste buds decrease in number and responsiveness. There is also a decrease in saliva production which contributes to dry mouth and tongue in the elderly.

Gradual structural changes occur in the kidney. Kidney function declines. The aging kidney responds more slowly and less efficiently in maintaining chemical balance in the body.

Bladder capacity decreases with age. Urgency may develop. Residual urine volume increases. Voiding sensation may be lessened. All of these changes may contribute to incontinence.

Research indicates that changes in the endocrine system include loss of receptor sites in target cells and decreased secretion from some glands. The consequences of these alterations are not known.

Cell loss in the brain occurs with aging. The effect of this cell loss is not clear. Neurons are not only lost but they also undergo change. Abnormal structures (plaques and tangles) develop in late life. Changes in neurotransmitter enzymes occur. Functional change involves a decrease in velocity of conduction of impulses resulting in the slowing of response time. This may be the underlying mechanism of many other changes seen in normal aging.

Sensory Changes

Some changes associated with aging have the potential for a major impact on health status. Sensory changes are in this category. Presbyopia results from changes in the lens and ciliary muscle. By age 50 corrective lens are needed almost universally for close work and reading (Botwinick, 1978). Visual acuity also declines as does the extent of the visual field. Dark adaptation and color vision also diminish. Cataract formation and glaucoma increase in incidence with age.

Health maintenance behaviors should include:

1. Regular examination by an opthalmologist;
2. Increasing the intensity of lighting for reading;
3. Using large print materials;
4. Scanning the environment frequently to prevent tripping;
5. Reducing glare by using matte finishes, shades, frosted bulbs and sun glasses;
6. Using night lights and florescent tape on switches;
7. Color coding medications with red or yellow not blue and green.

Hearing ability also declines with age. High pitched tones become less audible first. By age 60 presbycusis affects most people and serviceable hearing in the higher speech frequencies is lost (Botwinick, 1978). Consonants such as x, z, t, f, and g may become indiscriminable. Health maintenance behaviors required include:

1. Early audiometry testing to establish baseline data prior to presbycusis onset,
2. Periodic examination for cerumen buildup and removal as needed,
3. Attending to non-verbal cues,
4. Using artificial aids when needed,
5. Taking extreme care when driving or crossing streets,
6. Asking people to speak more slowly.

Sensitivity for all four basic tastes (salt, sweet, sour, bitter) declines after age 50. The ability to taste sweet is particularly affected by age (Goldman, 1979). This decline is related to a decrease in functioning taste buds and probably a decline in smell. Data available on the sense of smell is largely indirect or clinical in nature and thus less conclusive (Botwinick, 1978). Somatic sensations, including touch, pressure, vibration, position, and pain, decrease with age. Receptors become less sensitive and are fewer in number. Changes in taste, smell and touch also require the older person to develop protective behaviors. Some of these behaviors are:

1. Install smoke detectors,
2. Display reminders to turn off gas,
3. Monitor hot water temperature,
4. Use heating pads and hot water bottles cautiously,

5. Change position slowly,
6. Avoid over use of salt and sugar.

Decreased Mobility

Changes in joints, muscles, and the cardiovascular and nervous systems all contribute to decreased mobility in later years. Stiffness and decreased muscle tone and strength develop slowly. However, regular exercise can reduce the effects of aging on mobility. Lack of exercise can lead to premature aging (Birren & Sloane, 1980). Participating in a regular exercise program may be one of the most important things an elderly person can do to prepare for healthy aging. Recent studies have demonstrated that cardiac and pulmonary functioning and fitness improved over a six month period of regular exercise in elderly subjects (de Vries, 1980). Another study showed that state anxiety decreased in elderly subjects who exercised (Wiswell, 1980).

A basic exercise program should begin with a warm up of walking or jogging about one mile. The warm up should be followed by mild calisthenics aimed at moving all joints and strengthening large muscles. A cooling down period of stretches such as those used in yoga completes the program. This should be done at least three times a week. Isometric exercises are less desirable as they stimulate the vasovagal response, raising blood pressure.

One side effect of decreased mobility in later life is excess weight. As activity level goes down calorie consumption should also. Since basal metabolic rate also decreases with age, limiting intake is important to avoid excessive weight gain. Recommended dietary allowances for age 51 and over are 1800 calories for women and 2400 for men (Albanese, 1980).

Decreased mobility can also be a safety hazard for the elderly. Resting between activities, traveling at off peak hours, using handrails, removing scatter rugs, avoiding step ladders, putting rails on bathtubs and wearing sturdy shoes are all important preventive behaviors. Falls cause the highest number of accidents in the elderly, all too often leading to death (Houge, 1980).

Tissue Changes

Connective tissue and glandular changes described earlier in this paper require the elderly to take actions aimed at preventing irritation and ulcerations. The use of lubricants and moisturizers will help prevent cracking and peeling. Mild soaps should be used sparingly. The frequency of bathing may need to be decreased. Heavily perfumed cosmetics should be avoided. Gloves should be worn for housework. Older skin tans more easily; however, a good sun screen should be used to prevent drying. The development of age spots and some wrinkling cannot be prevented. Particular attention should be given to the feet. Trimming of nails and callouses should be done with extreme care or by a podiatrist. Careful drying between toes and prevention of blisters is important as decreased healing capacity may turn minor sores into major problems.

Changes in gastrointestinal tissue require careful attention to diet. Fluid intake must be maintained to prevent constipation or dehydration. Elderly people experiencing some problems with stress incontinence or frequency may try to avoid accidents by decreasing fluids. This should be discouraged. Instead, planning to assure regular access to toilet facilities or even the use of protective clothing are more effective ways of dealing with bladder problems. Adequate intake of roughage, fresh fruits, and vegetables and regular exercise will also assist digestion and elimination. Mild laxatives may be needed occasionally but the regular use of enemas or other electrolyte and energy depleting remedies should be avoided.

Changes in the oral cavity often result in denture use. Dentures should be removed for one to eight hours every day and should be brushed and stored in solution. Attention to oral hygiene is important to maintaining good nutrition and vice versa.

The mundane and relatively simple behaviors presented in this section need to be incorporated into the life style of the elderly to prevent disabilities arising from the physical changes related to the aging process. Psychosocial changes, especially those related to retirement, also require new behaviors to maintain health.

Psychosocial Changes

Research has demonstrated that there is no general decline in intelligence with age (Labouvie-Vief, 1979). However, there are changes in memory (Craik, 1977). Primary memory is not affected by age but secondary memory declines, probably due to a slowing in the CNS (central nervous system). Thus, both short and long term memory which require retrieval of material from storage are effected by age. Old people may appear to have good long term memories; however, the accuracy of their long term memory is poor in many instances. Preoccupation with the distant past may not be related to memory but rather to other psychological variables such as reminiscing.

Learning and problem solving abilities appear to decline with age. Memory may play a role in this decline. However, other significant factors are also involved. One factor is motivation. The older learner shows less motivation to learn material not directly related to an immediate need. The older learner is also more cautious in test situations. In fast paced testing, performance declines noticeably (Neugarten & Maddox, 1978). Anxiety may also interfere with learning. High levels of arousal have been demonstrated to occur more often in the elderly than in younger subjects and to interfere with learning (Eisdorfer, 1973). Concentration is another factor. The elderly are less able to ignore redundant or unimportant material when learning (Hoyer, Rebok, & Sued, 1979). Finally, society and the individual may expect poor performance, thus undermining self-esteem which can effect learning.

There is no convincing evidence that personality changes significantly with age (Schaie & Parham, 1976). Cognitive style, coping behaviors and self concept tend to remain the same as do personality traits (Thomae, 1981). Continuity theorists emphasize the stability of personality over time. Havighurst (1975) has identified eight personality types in old age. He suggests that these types are established by middle age and continue through old age.

Consistency of activity is also more common than marked change for the healthy aging individual. Thomae (1981) has reviewed and summarized studies of activity in the elderly. He concludes that activity is a complex trait. Types of activity may change with age and health status; however, degree of activity remains constant. The relationship of activity to morale is even more complex with many intervening variables. The most important of these is health status. Good health correlates with high morale regardless of activity level (Botwinick, 1978).

Developmental theorists describe changes that are universal, emphasizing tasks to be accomplished at various stages in life. Erikson's (1959) Stage VIII Ego Integrity versus Despair involves accepting one's life course, defending the dignity of one's life style and preparing for death. Others have identified the reinvestment of energy and attachment once associated with body image, occupation and sexuality as developmental tasks. New balances and perspectives related to dependency, aspiration and loss must be sought in late life (Zinberg & Kaufman, 1978). Butler (1975) has suggested that reminiscing on a ''Life Review'' is necessary to successful adjustment to aging. This process focuses attention on unresolved conflicts and may lead to resolution. Life review can be accompanied by nostalgia, anxiety and depression.

One change in behavior that was hypothesized in early studies to be a general characteristic of aging was an increase in introversion (Cameron, 1967). More recent studies have produced conflicting evidence (Schaie & Parham, 1976). No definitive statement concerning introversion as a characteristic of normal aging can be made at this time.

Other changes seen in many elderly include increased rigidity in some situations demanding change. This may be related to a decreased ability to problem solve and to a slowing of the CNS (Botwinick, 1978). A decrease in mastery over life is also experienced by many elderly, leading to lowered expectations and passivity. This seems to occur more frequently in men (Neugarten, 1964). Cautiousness and reluctance to take risks develops in many older persons; however, if risk taking is unavoidable then no age difference is demonstrated (Okun & Elias, 1977).

Role loss is a common experience for the elderly. Retirement, completion of the parental role, and widowhood precipitate role loss. Older people frequently maintain roles in voluntary associations if this has been a life long pattern. The role of friend is effected by the death of peers and movement to new communities. Some elderly increase their interactions with friends by moving to a retirement community. Proximity of age appropriate people is a critical factor in maintaining a social network (Kalish, 1975). Research indicates that having a close confidant is more important to satisfaction than the degree of social interaction (Lowenthal, 1967).

Retirement is a significant life event. There is no evidence that retirement itself effects health status (Haynes, McMichael, & Throyler, 1978). Most retirees adjust gradually to a new life style. To make this adjustment easier certain preventive actions should be taken. These include:

1. Preplanning to insure adequate income,
2. Developing friends not associated with work,
3. Tapering work in the last years before retirement by taking longer vacations, working shorter days or working part-time,

4. Developing daily routines to replace the structure of the work day,
5. Not relying on a spouse to fill all of the leisure time available,
6. Developing leisure time activities before retirement that are realistic in energy and monetary cost,
7. Preparing for exhilaration followed by disenchantment before a new satisfaction with one's life style develops,
8. Carefully assessing living arrangements, and if relocation is necessary, expending time in developing new social networks,
9. Expecting role loss to have a short term impact on self-esteem and one's marital relationship.

Changes in Sexuality

American society is just as ambivalent in its outlook toward sexuality as it is toward the aging process itself (Yoselle, 1981). Sexual behavior in late life may be inhibited by society's emphasis on youth, attractiveness, and efficiency. Further, society fosters the view that sexual activity is or should be beyond the scope and interest of the aging individual. In most instances this is not true. Sexual interest and capability continues throughout life.

Physical changes related to the aging process do effect sexual responsivity. Older individuals require higher levels of stimulation to achieve arousal. This may be related to changes in the CNS or to a decrease in fantasizing which occurs with aging (Cameron & Biba, 1973; Masters & Johnson, 1966). The capacity for orgasm declines in the older male but less so in the female. Secretions which provide lubrication during intercourse decline in the female. Vaginal tissues may become fragile after estrogen production ceases. Loss of a partner due to death or illness may change patterns and the frequency of sexual activity.

Actions which the elderly can take to maintain sexual activity include:

1. Regular stimulation through masturbation or intercourse to maintain elasticity in the female,
2. Use of lubrication or estrogen cream to decrease irritation,
3. Oral and digital manipulation to strengthen responses,
4. Avoidance of alcohol and medications prior to sex,
5. Pick a time of day when less tired and preparation time is adequate.

SERVICES REQUIRED TO SUPPORT HEALTH MAINTENANCE

Teaching and Counseling

Care providers in several professions and in many settings are in a position to provide teaching and counseling services for the elderly. Community groups, church groups, senior citizen centers, the workplace, adult education programs, health care centers are some of the potential settings available for classes, group sessions or individual counseling. In any setting guidelines for teaching and counseling the elderly should be observed. These include:

1. Use expanded speech (slow, spaced, clear),
2. Slow down non-verbal behavior,
3. Eliminate unnecessary detail,
4. Use brightly colored visuals,
5. Find quiet setting with good light,
6. Establish realistic goals,
7. Encourage group interaction,
8. Give positive feedback,
9. Encourage reminiscing,
10. Stimulate interest in building support network,
11. Support independence and active self care,
12. Build confidence and trust in care providers.

Screening/Referral

Screening programs need to be provided to separate the well from the at-risk. Early identification of those at-risk for the development of disabilities associated with aging can limit decline in function. Early detection of treatable pathology, often inappropriately attributed to the aging process, can often improve functioning. Programs should be designed to examine large numbers of elderly people in a short time period and at minimal cost. Such a program would include a health appraisal with elements such as vision and hearing testing, urinalysis, hematology, weight, physical and psychosocial status and health history.

A comprehensive screening program should also include outreach activities. Some elderly, for various reasons, will not attend screening sites. Efforts to locate these people in the community using mobile units, home visits and community members will improve the case finding potential of the program.

Referral to appropriate care providers and follow-up of referrals is the end result of the screening program. Obviously, close links to the teaching and counseling services discussed earlier are important to a good screening program. Alertness on the part of all care providers to the need for crisis intervention at any point in the process is necessary. The frequent losses associated with aging put this group at high risk for decreased self-esteem, depression and suicide. Prompt action to assist those in this category may be required.

Activity Oriented Services

Many of the health maintenance behaviors recommended in this paper involve activities for the elderly. Programs which make these activities accessible to the elderly are essential to prevention. Exercise programs, recreation programs, nutrition programs, and escort services are only some of the activities important to health maintenance in this age group. Provision of these services, along with the teaching, counseling, screening and referral services already described, is the responsibility of all care providers.

REFERENCES

Albanese, A. *Nutrition for the elderly.* New York: Alan R. Liss, 1980.

Behneke, J., Finch, C., & Moment, G., (Eds.). *The biology of aging.* New York: Plenum Press, 1978.

Binstock, R., & Shanas, E., (Eds.). *Handbook of aging and the social sciences.* New York: Von Nostrand Reinhold, 1976.

Birren, J., & Schaie, K.W., (Eds.). *Handbook of psychology of aging.* New York: Von Nostrand Reinhold, 1977.

Birren, J., & Sloane, R., (Eds.). *Handbook of mental health and aging.* Englewood Cliffs: Prentice-Hall, 1980.

Botwinick, J. *Aging and behavior,* (2nd ed.). New York: Springer, 1978.

Burnside, H. *Nursing and the aged,* (2nd ed.). New York: McGraw-Hill, 1981.

Busse, E.W., & Pfeiffer, E., (Eds.). *Behavior and adaptation in late life,* (2nd ed.). Boston: Little, Brown, 1977.

Butler, R., & Lewis, M. *Aging and mental health,* (2nd ed.). St. Louis: C.V. Mosby, 1977.

Butler, R. *Why survive? Being old in America.* New York: Harper and Row, 1975.

Cameron, P., & Biber, H. Sexual thought throughout the life-span. *Gerontologist,* 1973, *13,* 144-147.

Cameron, P. Introversion and egocentricity among the aged. *Journal of Gerontology,* 1967, *22,* 199-202.

Craik, F. Age differences in human memory. In J. Birren & K.W. Schaie (Eds.), *Handbook of psychology of aging.* New York: Von Nostrand Reinhold, 1977.

de Vries, H. Physiology of exercise and aging. In G. Lesnoff-Caravaglia (Ed.), *Health care of the elderly.* New York: Human Services Press, 1980.

Eisdorfer, C., & Lawton, M.P., (Eds.). *The psychology of adult development and aging.* Washington, D.C.: American Psychological Association, 1973.

Erikson, E. *Identity and the life cycle.* New York: Universities International Press, 1959.

Finch, C., & Hayflick, L., (Eds.). *Handbook of biology of aging.* New York: Von Nostrand Reinhold, 1977.

Gioiella, E., & Bevil, C. *Nursing care of the aging client.* New York: Appleton-Century-Crofts, in press.

Goldman, R. Decline in organ function with aging. In J. Rossman (Ed.), *Clinical geriatrics,* (2nd ed.). Philadelphia: J.B. Lippincott, 1979.

Havighurst, R. *Developmental tasks and education.* New York: David McKay, 1972.

Havighurst, R. Life styles transitions related to personality after age fifty. Paper presented at the International Society for Study of Behavioral Development Symposium, Kibbutz Kiravim, Israel, 1975.

Haynes, S., McMichael A., & Troyler, H. Survival after early and normal retirement. *Journal of Gerontology,* 1978, *33,* 269-278.

Hogue, C. Epidemiology of injury in older age. In *Epidemiology of aging.* Washington, D.C.: National Institutes of Health, 1980.

Kalish, R. *Late adulthood: Perspectives on human development.* Monterey, California: Brooks/Cole, 1975.

Lowenthal, M. Interaction and adaptation intimacy as a critical variable. *American Sociological Review,* 1968, *33,* 20-30.

Masters, W., & Johnson, V. *Human sexual response.* Boston: Little, Brown, 1966.

Neugarten, G., Crotley, W., & Tobin, S. *Personality in middle and late life.* New York: Atherton Press, 1964.

Neugarten, B., & Maddox, G. *Our future selves: A research plan toward understanding aging.* Washington, D.C.: National Institutes of Health, 1978.

Okun, M., & Elias, C. Cautiousness in adulthood as a function of age and payoff structure. *Journal of Gerontology,* 1977, *32,* 451-455.

Palmore, E., (Ed.). *Normal aging I and II.* Durham, N.C.: Duke University Press, 1974.

Rockstein, M. (Ed.). *Theoretical aspects of aging.* New York: Academic Press, 1974.

Rossman, I. (Ed.). *Clinical geriatrics,* (2nd ed.). Philadelphia: J.B. Lippincott, 1979.

Schaie, K., & Parham, I. Stability of adult personality traits: Facts or fable? *Journal of Personality and Social Psychology,* 1976, *34,* 146-158.

Shanas, E. Self-assessment of physical function in white and black elderly of the United States. In *Epidemiology of Aging.* Washington, D.C.: National Institutes of Health, 1980.

Siegel, J.S. Demographic aspects of aging and the older population in the United States. *Current population reports.* Washington, D.C.: United States Bureau of the Census, 1976.

Thomae, H. Personality and adjustment to aging. In J. Birren & R. Sloane (Eds.), *Handbook of mental health and aging.* Englewood Cliffs: Prentice-Hall, 1981.

Winick, M., (Ed.). *Nutrition and aging.* New York: John Wiley, 1976.

Wiswell, R. Relaxation, exercise and aging. In J. Birren & R. Sloane (Eds.), *Handbook of mental health and aging.* Englewood Clifs: Prentice-Hall, 1980.

Yoselle, H. Sexuality in the later years. *Topics in Clinical Nursing,* 1981, *3*(1), 59-70.

Yurick, H., Robb, S., Spier, B., & Ebert, N. *The aged person and the nursing process.* New York: Appleton-Century-Crofts, 1980.

Zinberg, N., & Kaufman, I. (Eds.). *Normal psychology of the aging process.* New York: International Universities Press, 1978.

Targeting Community Services to High-Risk Elders: Toward Preventing Long-Term Care Institutionalization

Alan M. Jette
Laurence G. Branch

ABSTRACT. Data from a probability sample of 1,625 elderly participants in the Massachusetts Health Care Panel Study were used to identify elders at high risk of long-term care (LTC) institutionalization. Advancing age, living alone, using assistance to perform basic and instrumental ADL, using an ambulation aid, and mental disorientation were significant predictors of entering a LTC facility during the six-year study period. A comparison of selected characteristics from the Massachusetts sample with a random sample of Massachusetts' Home Care Corporation recipients showed that the statewide approach to delivering home care successfully targeted services to high-risk elders. Future research should examine the extent to which targeting services to high-risk elders actually prevents or delays LTC institutionalization.

Long-term care (LTC) refers to the organization, financing, and delivery of a wide range of medical and social services to persons who are disabled or limited in their functional abilities over an extended period of time (Callahan & Wallach, 1981). Public support

---

Alan M. Jette is Assistant Professor of Gerontology and Physical Therapy at the MGH Institute of Health Professions, Assistant Professor of Social Medicine and Health Policy, and a member of the Division on Aging at Harvard Medical School.

Laurence G. Branch is a faculty member of Harvard Medical School and Harvard School of Public Health, a member of Harvard's Division on Aging, and a member of the Geriatric Research, Education, and Clinical Center at the Boston VA Outpatient Clinic. He is also the Director of the Massachusetts Health Care Panel Study.

This research was supported by grant number HS03815 from the National Center for Health Services Research, DHHS.

Address reprint requests to either author at Division on Aging, Harvard Medical School, 643 Huntington Avenue, Boston, MA 02115.

for LTC in the United States is heavily biased toward institutional care. Little public money is spent on LTC provided in the community relative to the amounts spent on nursing home care. Public financing for LTC comes primarily from Titles XVIII, XIX, and XX of the Social Security Act and Title III of the Older Americans Act. Medicaid, the major public source of LTC support, spent $211 million or only 1.2% of its $18 billion 1978 budget for home health care; it spent $7.2 billion or 40% of its budget for nursing home care. Medicare, on the other hand, devotes very little of its budget to any LTC. in 1979, for instance, Medicare spent only 1.3% of its $28 billion budget on nursing home care and 2.1% on home health care. Title XX allocated $530 million for homemaker or chore services in 1980, only 16% of its 2.7 billion dollar budget; while just 15% of Title III's $276 million 1980 allocation supported home health care (U.S. Government Accounting Office, 1981).

With so little public support of community-based LTC many elders with some LTC needs may be unnecessarily or inappropriately institutionalized in order to receive needed public support for their care. The U.S. Department of Health, Education & Welfare, for example, estimates that up to 25% of institutionalized patients could be cared for in less restrictive settings (U.S. Department of Health, Education & Welfare, 1978). A number of independent empirical studies support this estimate (U.S. Congressional Budget Office, 1977; Williams, Hill, Fairbank, & Knox, 1973).

A substantial degree of potentially unnecessary LTC institutionalization along with a major imbalance between the level of public support for institutional and community-based LTC have led many to recommend a major expansion in public support for noninstitutional LTC. Advocates defend this recommendation on economic as well as social or humanitarian grounds (Callahan & Wallach, 1981). A major barrier to this expansion is the fear that expanding the supply of noninstitutional LTC would result in an increased demand for noninstitutional care that would far surpass the decreased use of institutional services. Public officials fear that noninstitutional LTC, if expanded, would be used in addition to existing levels of institutional care and would not be used to prevent or postpone LTC institutionalization. An expanded publicly financed community LTC network that fails to reduce rates of LTC institutionalization could result either from decreasing use of informal sources of LTC support, generating new demand for LTC services among elders who had previously done without support, or both. If this occurs, it could lead to an enormous increase in society's LTC expenditures without reducing the use of institutional care.

Recent investigations provide some empirical basis for the fear that the goal of preventing unnecessary LTC institutionalization through the provision of noninstitutional services will be difficult to achieve. Hicks and her colleagues (1981) recently reported that patients who received coordinated home care services through project Triage had higher subsequent rates of LTC institutionalization than members of a matched comparison group who did not receive these services. In a randomized study of day care and home care services, Weissert and his associates (1979) found that while day care patients spent fewer days in skilled nursing facilities, day care probably served as an additional benefit under Medicare for the majority of patients rather than as a substitute for nursing home care. If our goal is to prevent the unnecessary use of institutional LTC we still face the challenge of developing effective ways of rectifying this institutional bias in LTC without drastically expanding the costs to our society.

Although many factors such as the level and type of informal home care support and the available supply of institutional services will ultimately influence whether the demand for institutional care can be reduced (Willemain, 1980), we contend that the goal of preventing unnecessary institutionalization can be reached by developing ways to identify and then successfully target noninstitutional LTC services to elders at high risk of institutionalization. We submit that a three step strategy will be required. First we need to develop means of identifying those elders who are at high risk of needing institutional care. The second step is to design programs that can target noninstitutional services to these high-risk elders. And finally we need to study whether or not targeting services to high-risk elders actually reduces the demand for institutional care.

Recent findings from two Massachusetts investigations shed light on the first two steps. Using data from the Massachusetts Health Care Panel Study (Branch & Fowler, 1975) new information is presented on risk factors for LTC institutionalization among the elderly. We also report on a recent investigation of the Massachusetts Home Care Corporation concept (Branch, 1979), a relatively recent large-scale attempt targeting community-based LTC services to high-risk elders. The key question of whether targeting community LTC to high-risk elders actually prevents LTC institutionalization remains to be addressed in future research.

RISK FACTORS FOR LTC INSTITUTIONALIZATION

A review of previous investigations of risk factors for LTC institutionalization confirms that it is by no means clear why some elders apply to or enter a LTC institution while others do not. Inspection of the results of these findings, as summarized in Table 1,

Table 1
Summary of Factors Related to LTC Institutionalization
in Seven Investigations

Characteristics	Townsend (1965)	Brody (1969)	Kraus (1976)	Brody (1978)	Greenberg (1979)	Neilson (1972)	Palmore (1976)
Demographic:							
Advanced Age	+	-	+	0	-	0	-
Not Married (single and/or widowed)	+	-	0	0	+	0	+
No Living Children	+	-	0	0	+	0	+
High Income	0	-	*	0	+	0	+
Lives Alone	0	-	+	+	-	+	+
Female	0	0	+	0	↓	0	-
White	0	0	0	0	0	0	+
Social:							
Socially Isolated	+	0	-	0	0	0	0
Lacks Social Support	+	0	*	+	+	0	0
Recent Loss of Social Support	+	0	0	0	-	0	0
Distance from Relatives	0	0	0	0	-	0	0
Functional Disability:							
Poor Health	0	-	+	0	0	0	0
Functional Disability	0	-	+	-	+	0	0
Multiple Problems	0	+	0	0	0	0	0
Multiple Medical Conditions	0	0	0	0	+	0	0
Unable to Take Medications	0	0	0	0	+	0	0
Unable to Prepare Meals	0	0	0	0	-	0	0
Attitudinal:							
Favorable Attitude Toward Institutionalization	0	+	0	0	+	0	0
Unable to Make Decisions	0	0	0	0	+	0	0
Lonely	0	0	+	0	-	0	0

+ = Characterizes institutionalized elders
* = Characterizes non-institutionalized elders
- = Does not differentiate
0 = The variable was not included in the study

illustrates that few of the variables studied are consistently related to LTC institutionalization.

Closer analysis of these studies reveals a number of potential reasons for these apparently discrepent results. There were major geographic differences in the populations studied. One sample came from Britain and Wales (Townsend, 1965); another consisted of Canadian elders (Krasu, Spasoff, Beattie, Holden, Lawson, Rodenburg, & Woodcock, 1976); the remaining samples came from the United States (Brody, 1969; Brody, 1978; Greenberg & Ginn, 1979; Nielsen, Blenkmer, Bloom, Downs, & Beggs, 1972; Palmore, 1976). In addition to these geographic differences, most of the investigations have limited generalizability since they examined nonprobability samples. The type of subjects also differed widely across the studies. Some compared applicants to LTC facilities with nonapplicants (Brody, 1969; Kraus et al., 1976); others compared residents of institutions with community elders (Townsend, 1965); still others compared LTC institutional residents with community elders using home care (Brody, 1978; Greenberg & Ginn, 1979; Nielsen et al., 1972). Except for the Greenberg and Ginn, and Palmore studies, all analyses were bivariate. The relative importance of each variable studied apropos the other variables in the analysis is unknown. And finally, most of the investigations were cross-sectional. Cross-sectional designs do not allow one to distinguish the effects of factors that may influence the decision to enter LTC institution from confounding factors such as the act of moving, the impact of institutionalization itself, or other unknown factors.

SAMPLE

The current investigation improved upon the shortcomings of previous research by employing a longitudinal, multivariate design with a statewide probability sample of elders. The data came from the first and third waves of the Massachusetts Health Care Panel Study (Branch & Fowler, 1975; Branch & Jette, 1982a). The original sample, drawn in late 1974, was a statewide probability sample of elders representative of the then noninstitutionalized population 65 years of age and older living in Massachusetts. Initial personal interviews were completed with 1,625 elders in early 1975, reflecting a 79% response rate from the initial pool of eligible respondents. The sample was almost excusively white (99%) and predominantly female (60%). The mean age of respondents in 1975 was 73 years. The demographic composition of the original sample was very similar to the 1970 census figures for noninstitutionalized elders in Massachusetts. Further details on the sampling procedures and the sample characteristics are available elsewhere (Branch & Jette, 1982b).

The original cohort was reinterviewed 15 months after the first contact. Since only a few elders had entered a LTC institution by that time, these analyses were postponed until the completion of the third wave. In late 1980 the cohort was contacted for the third time. Of the initial 1,625 participants, 825 (51%) were reinterviewed; 416 (25%) had died in the ensuing six years; 4% were then residing in a LTC institution; 13% were recontacted but refused to continue their participation; 2% had moved out of Massachusetts or were temporarily absent and therefore not interviewed; and 5% could not be located.

Since approximately 20% of the original cohort were lost to follow-up during the six-year study, attrition could be a potential limitation to this study. To examine the implications of this attrition rate, the age, gender, living situation, and use of assistance in ADL as determined in the initial 1975 interview for those lost to follow-up were compared with the 825 elders interviewed in 1980. No statistically significant differences in those characteristics were found across the two groups. The confidence in generalizing these findings to the population of elders living in Massachusetts is therefore increased.

STUDY VARIABLES

In this analysis, nursing homes and chronic disease hospitals were considered LTC institutions. Thus defined, 147 elders, 9% of the original cohort, entered a LTC institution sometime during the six-year study period. This included 60 elders who were in a LTC institution at the time of the third interview, 69 elders who died in a LTC institution, and 18 who entered a LTC institution but were subsequently discharged back to the community. Information on LTC institutionalization was collected by project field staff (i.e., from the personal interview or from attempts to recontact a respondent) and from death certificates which listed the place of death. A respondent was considered institutionalized regardless of length of stay in the LTC institution. Thus, individuals who stayed in a LTC institution only for a brief period prior to death were included in this analysis. Missing from this categorization were those who died during the interim and who had been in an LTC institution during the study but died either in an acute care hospital or in the community after being released from the LTC institution. Excluding these individuals from the following analysis does not limit the generalizability of the findings, but does limit using the 9% figure as a six-year incidence rate.

The explanatory power of six socio-demographic and seven disability variables was examined. These variables were selected from those identified as potential predictors in previous research. All predictors were constructed from information collected in the 1975 interview. The socio-demographic predictors include respondents' age, gender, education, Medicaid eligibility, living situation, and marital status. Respondents' age, gender, and education are taken directly from the personal interview. Medicaid eligibility is a binary variable which defines eligibility as living alone with an annual income in 1974 of less than $5,000 or living with someone else with a joint annual income of less than $7,000. Living situation categorizes respondents living alone or living with other people; the marital status variable separates the widowed from respondents in all other marital states.

The seven disability indices include an assessment of sight deficit, hearing acuity, gross functional disability, use of ambulation aids, mental orientation, use of assistance in basic activities of daily living (ADL), and use of assistance in instrumental ADL. Sight deficit was determined by respondents' report of whether they see well enough to read newspaper or magazine print (with corrective lenses if necessary). Hearing acuity represents respondents' perceptions of the quality of their hearing (with hearing aids if necessary). Gross functional disability categorizes respondents who report having a physical health problem which bothers them or who are unable to do heavy work, climb stairs, or walk a half mile. Use of ambulation aids identifies those elders who use a walker or wheel chair. Mental orientation is the interviewer's subjective judgment of the respondent's degree of orientation at the time of the initial interview. The use of assistance in basic ADL identifies elders who use mechanical or human assistance in performing one or more of six basic ADL: walking, transferring, dressing, bathing, eating, and grooming. Use of assistance in instrumental ADL identifies those who use assistance from another person in housekeeping, transportation, food preparation or grocery shopping.

MAJOR RISK FACTORS

Table 2 displays the means, standard deviations, and pairwise correlations of all variables used in this analysis. All nominal variables were converted to dummy variables. Stepwise logistic regression was used to estimate the predictive power of these 13 independent variables on subsequent LTC institutionalization. The procedure uses maximum likelihood estimates computed by the Newton-Raphson method. This procedure provides a Model Chi square, a Model D statistic (comparable to R^2), and individual variable d statistics (partial R^2) in addition to betas and standard errors.

Table 3 displays the six key variables which achieve significant correlation with LTC institutionalization. Advancing age, living alone, using ambulation aids, mental disorientation, and using assistance to perform basic or instrumental ADL all significantly increase the risk of LTC institutionalization. This regression model achieves a predictive accuracy coefficient of .59 with $D = 0.093$. To further elucidate key risk factors for subsequent institutionalization, a second regression was calculated which includes first-order interaction terms in the model. When interaction terms are included, younger elders who live alone, older respondents who use assistance in instrumental ADL, and disoriented elders living with other people are significantly more likely to enter a LTC institution. This regression model with interaction effects increased slightly the explanatory power of the predictive variables.

TARGETING HOME CARE SERVICES
TO HIGH-RISK ELDERS

Having presented some empirical findings which identify characteristics of elders at high risk of entering a LTC institution, the investigation turns to the second issue of how one might target home care services to these high-risk groups (Branch, 1979; Branch, Callahan, & Jette, 1981). Once high-risk elders are identified can community services be targeted to them?

One innovative approach to community LTC has been in operation in Massachusetts for the past decade. In 1973, the Massachusetts' Department of Elder Affairs began to establish Home Care Corporations (HCC) to deliver home care services to elders in each of 27 service areas located around the state. The first two HCCs

Table 2

Pairwise Correlations, Means, and Standard Deviations of Variables Used in Analysis

	(n)	1	2	3	4	5	6	7	8	9	10	11	12	13	14
1. Age	(1619)	1.0													
2. Gender	(1625)	-.03	1.0												
3. Education	(1566)	-.17	.00	1.0											
4. Medicaid Eligible	(1625)	.02	.04	-.24	1.0										
5. Lives Alone	(1624)	-.11	.21	-.06	-.22	1.0									
6. Widowed	(1615)	-.27	.33	.09	.10	.48	1.0								
7. Assistance in Basic ADL	(1625)	.21	-.14	-.07	.00	.05	.12	1.0							
8. Assistance in Instrumental ADL	(1625)	.13	.20	-.13	.01	-.41	-.19	.12	1.0						
9. Sight Deficit	(1609)	.18	-.04	-.13	-.02	-.04	.07	.18	.09	1.0					
10. Hearing Acuity	(1600)	.23	.06	-.18	.10	-.02	.05	.11	.10	.12	1.0				
11. Functional Disability	(1625)	.29	-.11	-.22	.08	-.02	.11	.42	.22	.26	.24	1.0			
12. Ambulation Aid	(1623)	.19	-.07	-.07	.03	.03	.12	.26	.09	.15	.08	.33	1.0		
13. Mental Orientation	(1579)	-.10	-.03	.01	.04	.05	.03	-.08	-.06	-.13	-.03	-.11	.03	1.0	
14. LTC Institutionalization	(1305)	.27	-.04	-.06	.06	.10	.11	.16	.07	.09	.09	.18	.17	-.12	1.0
Mean		2.3	1.4	6.7	0.5	0.3	0.4	0.3	0.8	0.1	2.1	0.3	0.1	1.9	0.1
Standard Deviation		1.2	0.5	3.5	0.5	0.4	0.5	0.5	0.4	0.2	0.8	0.3	0.2	0.1	0.3
Percentage of Dichotomous Variables		-	1=60 2=40	-	0=54 1=46	0=72 1=28	0=63 1=37	0=69 1=31	0=23 1=77	0=94 1=6	-	-	0=97 1=3	0=2 1=98	0=91 1=9

Discrete Variable Values: Age: 1=65-69, 2=70-74, 3=75-79, 4=80-84, 5=85+ yrs.; Gender: 1=female, 2=male; Education: 1=no formal education...13=graduate school; Medicaid Eligible: 0=no, 1=yes; Lives Alone: 0=no, 1=yes; Widowed: 0=no, 1=yes; Assistance in Basic ADL: 0=no, 1=yes; Assistance in Instrumental ADL: 0=no, 1=yes; Sight Deficit: 0=no, 1=yes; Hearing Acuity: 1=excellent, 2=good, 3=fair, 4=poor; Uses Ambulation Aid: 0=no, 1=yes; Mental Orientation: 0=disoriented, 1=oriented; LTC Institutionalization: 0=no, 1=yes.

Table 3

Stepwise Logistic Regression of Risk Factors of
Long-Term Care Institutionalization

Risk Factors	Beta	Standard Error	d
Age	0.46**	0.08	0.03
Lives Alone	0.98**	0.23	0.02
Uses Ambulation Aid	1.36**	0.39	0.01
Mental Disorientation	1.30**	0.49	0.01
Uses Assistance in Basic ADL	0.52*	0.22	0.01
Uses Assistance in Instrumental ADL	0.65*	0.31	0.00
N	(1121)		
Predictive Accuracy Coefficient	0.59		
D Statistic (R-squared)	0.093**		
Model Chi-Square	121 with 6 df		

*$p < .05$
**$p < .001$

were established in 1973; all 27 service areas were covered by July of 1977.

The Massachusetts approach to delivering home care was based upon six concepts.

1. *Destigmatization.* Home care services are not provided through the Department of Public Welfare under the Old Age Assistance Program. It was hoped that removing home care services from the welfare model would destigmatize them, thus opening up the possibility for more people to apply for the services they might need.

2. *Local consumer/input.* Elders at the local level are directly involved in policy making and decision making. This approach reflects the assumption that a truly responsive home care program must consider local needs from the perspective of older individuals.

3. *Minimization of red tape.* The program seeks to avoid the well known problems of bureaucratic red tape, including civil service and state purchasing requirements, in the interest of facilitating the provision of services to the elderly.

4. *Case management.* Home care services are targeted to elders with a combination of needs who require a multiplicity of services, frequently from many agencies. To overcome the difficult process of traveling through the labyrinth of multiple service agencies, the Massachusetts home care model includes strong case management as a key element. The older person's needs are assessed in one location for a variety of services.

5. *Multiple funding.* Funds for services to the elderly come from a variety of sources including Titles XVIII, XIX, and XX of the Social Security Act and Title III of the Older Americans Act. A package of services, complete with all the funding arrangements, can be authorized on behalf of the older person.

6. *Priority to the elderly.* The fact that some service agencies discriminate against the elderly has been documented (U.S. Commission on Civil Rights, 1977). Thus Massachusetts created an agency uniquely designed for the elderly to avoid the possibility of age discrimination.

To what extent is this Massachusetts HCC approach able to target services to elders at high risk of subsequent LTC institutionalization? This question was addressed empirically by comparing some of the demonstrated high-risk characteristics of the HCC clients with the characteristics of a statewide sample of elders. It was hypothesized that if the HCCs were targeting services successfully to a high-risk group, a substantially larger portion of HCC recipients would have these high-risk characteristics compared with their distribution in a probability sample of noninstitutionalized elders living in Massachusetts.

METHOD

In November, 1978, 302 HCC recipients were randomly selected from the 22,941 active recipients from all 27 HCCs. Of these, 16 were ineligible for the study because their cases had been closed for legitimate reasons (e.g., death, temporary relocation, hospitalization, etc.). Of the 286 remaining eligible recipients, 251 (88%) agreed to participate in the study and completed a personal interview. Included in this personal interview were three high-risk factors identified in our longitudinal analyses: chronological age, living situation, and use of instrumental ADL.

To examine the extent to which HCCs are targeting services to high-risk elders a comparison was made of the distribution of age, living situation, and use of instrumental ADL assistance in the HCC recipient sample with the distribution in a probability sample of non-institutionalized elders aged 65 or older living in Massachusetts. Data on the statewide samples came from Branch's second wave of the Massachusetts Health Care Panel Study (Branch, 1977). The chi-square statistic was used to determine the statistical significance of differences between the two groups.

RESULTS

As Table 4 indicates, a significantly larger proportion of the HCC recipients as compared to the statewide elderly population were of advanced age and lived alone. Only 31% of the HCC sample were under 75 years of age compared with 60% of Massachusetts elders. Twenty percent of HCC recipients were 85 years or older while only 7% of the statewide sample were members of this oldest age cohort. Seventy-one percent of the HCC recipients lived alone compared to 30% of the statewide sample.

Table 5 further illustrates that the HCC are targeting services to

Table 4

Comparison of the Age and Living Situation of
Home Care Corporation Recipients with a
Massachusetts Sample of Elders

Characteristic	HCC Recipients	Massachusetts Sample	
Age:			
65-74 years	31%	60%	
75-84 years	49	33	$\chi^2(2)=85*$
85+ years	20	7	
(N)	(244)	(1311)	
Living Situation:			
Alone	71	30	
With Spouse and/or Children	24	55	$\chi^2(2)=153*$
Other Combinations	5	15	
(N)	(251)	(1317)	

*p< .001

Table 5

Comparison of Self-Sufficiency in Instrumental ADL
of Home Care Corporation Recipients with a
Massachusetts Sample of Elders

Instrumental ADL	HCC Recipients			Massachusetts Sample			
	(N)	Self-Sufficient	Not Self-Sufficient	(N)	Self-Sufficient	Not Self-Sufficient	
Housekeeping	(250)	11%	89%	(1289)	51%	49%	$\chi^2(1)=136$*
Transportation	(231)	11	89	(1290)	56	44	$\chi^2(1)=159$*
Grocery Shopping	(248)	39	61	(1302)	61	39	$\chi^2(1)=41$*
Food Preparation	(232)	60	40	(1286)	61	39	$\chi^2(1)=-.08$

*p<.001

elders with instrumental activity needs. Significantly larger proportions of HCC recipients compared to the total statewide elderly sample were *not* self-sufficient in housekeeping, transportation, and grocery shopping. Food preparation was the only instrumental ADL in which a similar proportion of elders in the two groups used assistance.

In all cases where risk factors are available, except for food preparation, the HCC sample appears to be at greater risk of institutionalization than the statewide sample.

DISCUSSION

Findings from these two investigations clarify two important issues with respect to preventing LTC institutionalization. Analyses of the Massachusetts Health Care Panel data provide preliminary support for the proposition that elders at high risk of entering a LTC institution can be identified empirically. The Massachusetts HCC experience suggests that home-based LTC services can be targeted to these high-risk groups. Such results are encouraging evidence for those who believe that current rates of LTC institutionalization may be reduced by targeting noninstitutional services to high-risk individuals.

Albeit encouraging, these findings are only a beginning. A large proportion of the total variance in LTC institutionalization remains unexplained by this investigation. Furthermore, the key question still to be addressed is whether or not targeting home care services to high-risk elders actually prevents or delays LTC institutionalization. Some argue that targeting services to high-risk groups is a poor way of using scarce home care resources (Willemain, 1980). Recent empirical investigations, in fact, suggest that providing home care services to elders may not reduce the rate of LTC institutionalization. These investigations, however, did not target services to high-risk elders. In the Weissert et al. investigation (1979), for example, participants were Medicare-eligible elders referred by health care providers and social service agencies. Inspection of the study population characteristics shows that, in contrast to the type of clients served by the Massachusetts HCC, over half of their day care experimental group were under 75 years of age, while only 23% lived alone. It would be interesting to examine whether or not rates of institutionalization were reduced for high-risk subgroups within this experimental population. A similar picture emerges when one examines the sample characteristics in the Triage investigation (Hicks et al., 1981). To be eligible for this demonstration the individual had to be over 60 years of age, Medicare-eligible, and a resident of a specific geographic region. Forty percent of the Triage study population were under 75 years of age and only 34% lived alone.

Future investigations aimed at preventing LTC institutionalization need to focus on high-risk groups of elders to examine if targeting services to those at risk of entering a LTC institution will prevent or delay subsequent institutionalization. Only then can one know if programs like the Massachusetts HCCs are successful in preventing or delaying LTC institutionalization.

The Massachusetts Health Care Panel Study analyses further illustrate that risk of entering a LTC institution involves many facother than an elder's physical impairment. These findings reveal that risk, at least in this population, is influenced by advancing age, living alone, and mental disorientation, as well as by dependence in ADL. Home care designed to prevent LTC institutionalization should be targeted to elders with these characteristics or other risk factors not yet identified. The type of home care needed by these elders to reduce their risk of LTC institutionalization remains to be addressed in other studies. Promising work is currently in progress on this important question (Sager, 1982).

Only 13% of the variance in LTC institutionalization was explained by the Massachusetts Health Care Panel Study data. There are many potential reasons for this limited explanatory power. The most obvious explanation might be that LTC institutionalization is influenced primarily by an elder's medical condition. The Massachusetts Health Care Panel Study has a limited scope, using only respondent self-report measures, which precludes the most reliable examination of specific diseases and pathological conditions which may have a major impact on LTC institutionalization. Events or conditions not present at the start of the Massachusetts Health Care Panel Study that occurred during the intervening years are also excluded from our analyses. Other factors such as the supply of LTC beds, attitudinal and other psychosocial variables, and various situational characteristics are also absent from these analyses. Finally, missing from the categorization of having entered a LTC institution are those who died in an acute care hospital or in the community after being released from a LTC institution. Future research needs to improve upon these shortcomings in order to develop a more comprehensive and consistent body of knowledge about key factors influencing elder's risk of LTC institutionalization.

These preliminary analyses of the Massachusetts HCC model are instructive in other ways as well. The HCC approach is one of the first statewide networks in the United States trying to deliver and coordinate home care services to elders. It operates independent of the medical model used in programs such as Medicare where access to home care is based on medical need. The HCC program operates under nonprofit auspices and involves consumers at the local level in policymaking. We are encouraged by these findings which clearly illustrate that this program is reaching its intended target group: those elders shown empirically to be at high risk of entering a LTC institution. The precise elements of the Massachusetts program that contribute to its success cannot be determined from these data. This remains to be addressed by future research.

REFERENCES

Branch, L. G. *Understanding the health care needs of people over age 65*. Boston, MA: Center for Survey Research Monograph, University of Massachusetts and the Joint Center for Urban Studies of M.I.T. and Harvard University, 1977.

Branch, L. G. *Who are the home care corporation Title XX recipients in Massachusetts*. Boston, MA: Center for Survey Research, University of Massachusetts and the Joint Center for Urban Studies of M.I.T. and Harvard University, 1979.

Branch, L. G., Callahan, J. J., & Jette, A. M. Targeting home care services to vulnerable elders: Massachusetts' home care corporations. *Home Health Care Services Quarterly*. 1981, *2*(2), 41-58.

Branch, L. G., & Fowler, F. J. *The health care needs of the elderly and chronically disabled in Massachusetts*. Boston, MA: Center for Survey Research Monograph, University of Massachusetts and the Joint Center for Urban Studies of M.I.T. and Harvard University, 1975.

Branch, L. G., & Jette, A. M. *The Massachusetts health care panel study: Third wave descriptive findings*. Boston, MA: Division on Aging Monograph, Harvard Medical School, 1982(a).

Branch, L. G., & Jette, A. M. A prospective study of long-term care institutionalization among the aged. *American Journal of Public Health,* in press, 1982 (b).

Brody, E. Follow-up study of applicants and non-applicants to a voluntary home. *Gerontologist,* 1969, *9*, 187-196.

Brody, S., Poulshock S., & Masciocchi, C. The family caring unit: A major consideration in the long-term support system. *Gerontologist*, 1978, *18*, 556-561.

Callahan, J. J., & Wallack, S. S. *Reforming the long-term care system*. Lexington, MA: Lexington Books, 1981.

Greenberg, J., & Ginn, A. A multivariate analysis of the predictors of long-term care placement. *Home Health Care Services Quarterly*, 1979, *1*, 75-99.

Hicks, B., Raisz, H., Segal, J., & Doherty, N. The triage experiment in coordinated care for the elderly. *American Journal of Public Health*, 1981, *71*, 991-1003.

Kraus, A., Spasoff, R., Beattie, E., Holden, E., Lawson, S., Rosenburg, M., & Woodcock, G. Elderly applicants to long-term care institutions I. Their characteristics: Health problems and state of mind. *Journal of the American Geriatric Society,* 1976, *24,* 117-125.

Nielsen, M., Blenkmer, M., Bloom, M., Downs, T., & Beggs, H. Older persons after hospitalization: A controlled study of home aide service. *American Journal of Public Health,* 1972, *62,* 1094-1101.

Palmore, E. Total chance of institutionalization among the aged. *Gerontologist,* 1976, *16,* 504-507.

Sager, A. Evaluating the home care service needs of the elderly. *Home Health Care Services Quarterly,* 1982, *3,* 81-85.

Townsend, P. The effects of family structure on the likelihood of admission to an institution in old age: The application of a general theory. In E. Shanas & G. Streib, (Eds.), *Social structure and the family.* Englewood Cliffs: Prentice-Hall, 1965.

U.S. Congressional Budget Office. *Long-term care for the elderly and disabled.* Washington, D.C.: U.S. Government Printing Office, 1977.

U.S. Commission on Civil Rights. *The age discrimination study.* Washington, D.C.: U.S. Government Printing Office, 1977.

U.S. Department of Health, Education & Welfare. *Program design choices for long-term care legislative initiatives-decision memorandum.* Washington, D.C., 1974.

U.S. Department of Health, Education & Welfare. *Major Initiative: Long-Term Care/Community Services.* Office of the Secretary, Briefing memorandum, Washington, D.C., July 14, 1978.

U.S. General Accounting Office. *Improved knowledge base would be helpful in reaching policy decisions on providing long-term in-home services for the elderly* (HRD-82-4). Report to the Honorable Pete V. Domenici, United States Senate, Washington, D.C., 1981.

Weissert, W., Wan, T., & Livieratos, B. *Effects and costs of day care and homemaker services for the chronically ill: A randomized experiment* (DHEW Pub. No. PHS 79-3250). Washington, D.C.: National Center for Health Services Research, 1979.

Willemain, T. R. Beyond the GAO Cleveland study: Client selection for home care services. *Home Health Care Services Quarterly,* 1980, *1,* 65-83.

Williams, T. F., Hill, J. G., Fairbank, M. E., & Knox, K. G. Appropriate placement of the chronically ill & aged. *Journal of the American Medical Association,* 1973, *226*(11), 1332-1335.

Prevention of Unnecessary Geriatric Deaths: Differential Rate of Morbidity/Mortality on Admission to Long Term Care Facilities

Helen West

ABSTRACT. The amount of trauma experienced by elderly entering nursing homes appears to be a function of a number of environmental factors. The present study uses physician visits, PRN medication requests, the number of prescription medications administered, and mortality to compare the effects of two nursing home types, nonprofit and proprietary, on the elderly over a period of seven months. Physician visits, medication requests, and the number of prescription medications administered fluctuated in the nonprofit homes over the seven months while they decreased and then stabilized in the proprietary homes. Mortality was significantly higher in the proprietary homes. The implications of these findings for preventive interventions are discussed.

The trauma of entry into a nursing home has been assessed in various geriatric populations. A number of studies have reported on specific psychological and physiological effects which the aged experience as a result of radical environmental change (Bourestom, Pastalan, & Tars, 1973; Fried, 1963; Friedsom, 1962; Lawton & Yaffe, 1967; Miller, 1965). Effects appear to vary as a function of several, perhaps interactive variables. Lieberman, Prack, and Tobin (1968) posit that many negative effects ascribed to institutionalization are related to the decision to enter the institution. In other words, the decline in well being associated with relocation to an in-

Reprints may be requested from Helen West, Gerontology Services Administration, University of Texas Health Science Center, 5323 Harry Hines Boulevard, Dallas, TX 75235.

stitution may begin immediately prior to actual entrance. The extent to which entry is voluntary seems to be another factor which influences subsequent vulnerability (Farrari, 1963; Schulz & Aderman, 1973; Turner, Tobin, & Lieberman, 1972). Some relocation studies suggest that interinstitutional transfer may not produce increased morbidity or mortality (Dobson & Patterson, 1961; Epstein & Simon, 1967; Stotsky, 1967); instead, such a move may result in an enhancement of positive affect (Donahue, 1965; Goldfarb, Shahinian, & Turner, 1966). However, the change from community living to institutional living appears to be accompanied by increased morbidity and/or mortality (Aldrich & Mendkoff, 1963; Goldfarb et al., 1966; Jasnau, 1967; Lieberman, 1961). One study of relocation from home to an institution showed the death rate was two and one-half times greater than in the waiting period before entry (Lieberman, Tobin, & Slover, 1971). When the entry is to a physically superior or preferable setting, length of life may be increased and the usual high death rate diminished (Ogren & Linn, 1971). The same is true when appropriate environmental alteration and adequate staff training are affected (Stotsky, 1970).

Lieberman (1969) suggests that the study of "psychological loss" may offer an effective model for identifying factors leading to the noxious effects of institutionalization. He suggests one primary consideration is the relationship between pre- and post-relocation environments. For instance, relocation to environments which limit self-regulation, relative to the previous environment, may be highly stressful (Aldrich & Mendkoff, 1963; Kral, Grad, & Berenson, 1968; Markus, Blenker, Bloom, & Downs, 1971, 1972; Miller & Lieberman, 1965). Moreover, when the individual leaves a familiar and well-liked environment (Barton, 1962; Killian, 1970), giving up clothing and personal items (Schoenberg, Carr, Peretz, & Kutscher, 1970), excess stress and depression may result. Even relocation within the immediate physical environment can be stressful when social interaction patterns are disrupted (Sommer & Ross, 1958). Alternatively, if the post-relocation environment contains the rewards and opportunities for self-regulation, psychological warmth, informal contacts and friends, then relocation may be less stressful (Burgess, 1954; Messer, 1968; Michelson, 1954). In other words, it seems that the critical factor is radical environmental change involving psychological/social loss rather than the fact of institutionalization per se.

These studies seem to suggest there are major differences in the institutions to which patients are admitted. Some may have superior environments, better educated staff, and more opportunity for self-regulation, individualization, and psychological warmth. The implication is that these factors affect the morbidity/mortality associated with entry.

Categorization of institutions is usually done on the basis of ownership. Proprietary homes constitute the largest number of homes in the country and outnumber not-for-profit (usually church supported) homes more than two to one (Pegels, 1981). There has been criticism of this development to the effect that government policy encourages the predominance of economic considerations over patient care needs (U.S. Congress, Senate, Special Committee on Aging, 1971). This presumed difference in the quality of care related to type of facility has been studied by Levey, Kinlock, Stotsky, Ruchlin, and Oppenheim (1971) who noted no significant difference in quality of care by type of ownership. In this study, quality of care was identified as compliance with selected characteristics in nine major areas: nursing service, dietary service, restorative services, patient activities, physical plant, physician's order book, nursing kardex, patient records, and personal care of the patient. Anderson, Holmberg, and Stone (1967) reported that interactional qualities of how a facility is administrated seem to explain variation in quality of care better than structural variables, including ownership. However, it remains for overall quality to be measured directly in relation to the impact on residents (Sherwood, 1975). This study was designed to assess differential rates of mortality and approximations of morbidity in a representative sample of proprietary and nonprofit nursing homes beds, using patient impact measures.

METHOD

A stratified sample of nursing home beds was selected to reflect the differential proportion of not-for-profit to proprietary beds in a large urban area. The sample number of beds (N = 555) accounted for 17% of the total number of beds in the area. Two hundred and nine beds represented the strata of not-for-profit homes and 346 beds represented the strata of proprietary homes. Facilities were randomly selected for study from a pool of clinical affiliates with the University of Texas Health Science Center at Dallas. The pool was first dichotomized between proprietary and nonprofit facilities. Five homes provided a properly stratified sample, reflecting The Profile of the Texas Area 5 Health Systems agency long term care facilities inventory. These long term care facilities represented a mix of Intermediate Care beds and Skilled Nursing beds. Beds so designated refer to the type of medical needs prospective occupants may have and are filled as a result of specific level of care evaluation. All patients who had entered these facilities for nursing care at month one of the study became the research population and were followed for seven months.

Morbidity was approximated by measuring the number of physician visits, the number of requests for PRN medications, and the number of prescription medications administered. Mortality rates were counted over the same period.

RESULTS

Analysis of variance was used to determine significant differences in measures of physician visits, PRN medications, prescription medications and mortality rates over time. Follow-up analyses were performed using the Newman-Keuls technique for identifying where significant differences occurred without sacrificing the .05 level of confidence in the findings (Huck, Cormier, & Bounds, 1974). In the combined sample, physician visits decreased significantly between the first two months, with no significant variability thereafter (.05 was utilized as the level of confidence in all analyses). PRN medications were requested significantly fewer times from month 1 to 2 with no change noted from month 2 to 3. A significant decrease occurred again from month 3 to 4, and no significant change was noted thereafter. Prescription medications were administered significantly fewer times between month 1 and 2, and between month 2 and 3, but there was no change in frequency between month 3 and 4. A significant decrease occurred between month 4 and 5, but no significant changes were noted in the remaining months studies (Fig. 1).

In the not-for-profit sample, physician visits decreased significantly from month 1 to 2, remained unchanged from month 2 to 3, increased significantly between month 3 and 4, decreased significantly from month 4 to 5, and showed no change in frequency from month 5 to 6, but increased significantly from month 6 to 7. The frequency of PRN medications administered decreased significantly

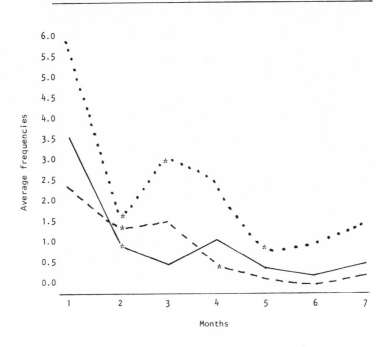

Fig. 1. Frequency of Measures of Morbidity in the
Combined Not-For-Profit and Proprietary Groups

*Means are significantly different from previous month, p < .05.

Physician visits (————)
Prescription medications (• • • •)
PRN medications (- - - -)

from month 1 to 2, increased significantly from month 2 to 3, decreased significantly from month 3 to 4 and again from month 4 to 5, remained the same from month 5 to 6 and increased significantly from month 6 to 7. The prescription medications administered in this group decreased significantly from month 1 to 2, increased significantly from month 2 to 3, remained the same from month 3 to 4, decreased significantly from month 4 to 5, were unchanged from month 5 to 6, and increased significantly from month 6 to 7 (Fig. 2).

In the proprietary sample the physician visits decreased significantly from month 1 to 2 and remained without significant variance from months 2 through 7. The administration of PRN medications decreased significantly from month 1 to 3 and showed no more sig-

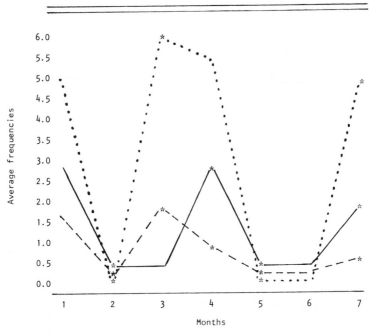

Fig. 2. Frequency of Measures of Morbidity in the Not-For-Profit Group

*Means are significantly different from previous month, p < .05.

Physician visits (————)
Prescription medications (• • • •)
PRN medications (- - - -)

nificant variability from months 3 to 7. The frequency of prescription medications administered decreased significantly from month 1 to 2 with no significant variance thereafter (Fig. 3).

Death rates showed no statistically significant difference within either group over time. However, a chi square test for independence between not-for-profit and proprietary beds sampled showed significantly fewer deaths in the not-for-profit group than in the proprietary group (Table 1).

DISCUSSION

When the data are analyzed separately by type of facility, there seems to be a linear relationship between measures approximating morbidity and length of time from entry in the proprietary beds during the first two months. Subsequent months show no significant fluctuation over the time of the study. Figure 3 indicates the significance of changes in frequency of these measures in the proprietary subjects. The significance of changes in the same measures of subjects in the not-for-profit facilities cannot be represented by a linear relationship, suggesting some factors germane to the not-for-profit nursing home may have an ameliorative influence in entry-associated morbidity (Fig. 2). The assumption of beneficial influence is based on the significant difference in death rates between the two sample groups. Prevention of unnecessary deaths may be related to the differential response in care giving occurring in such facilities. Table 1 shows comparative rates of mortality over time for each sample.

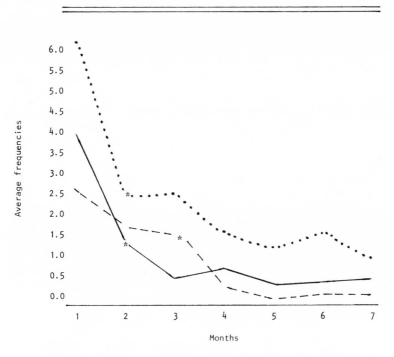

Fig. 3. Frequency of Measures of Morbidity in the Proprietary Group

*Means are significantly different from the previous month, p < .05.

Physician visits (————)
Prescription medications (• • • •)
PRN medications (- - - -)

Table 1

2 X 2 Contingency Table for Deaths by Sample Groups

	Dead	Alive	
Not-For-Profit	3	17	20
Proprietary	23	34	57
	26	51	77

$x^2 = 3.84$, $p < .05$

The findings in this study appear to indicate the need for hasty intervention at the time of entry into a nursing home in order to prevent unnecessary fatalities. In the proprietary sample, morbidity indicators and death rates show an unmatched frequency the first month, followed by a progressive decline. This type of facility accounts for 77% of nursing home beds, clearly the great majority (Pegels, 1981). The fact that the not-for-profit sample showed no such pattern may be related to any one of a number of factors. One possibilities is that care (in terms of medications and physicians' visits) reflects a closely monitored response to patient need and therefore fluctuates idiosyncratically. It is also possible that other factors such as those identified in previous studies (Burgess, 1975; Messer, 1968; Michelson, 1954) have a preventive effect on an otherwise general pattern of decline. If so, perhaps these factors are present to a greater extent in not-for-profit environments. Thus unnecessary morbidity and mortality is prevented.

CONCLUSIONS

In order to prevent untimely geriatric deaths precipitated by the trauma associated with institutionalization, some approaches are suggested by this study. Since in the majority of cases, the greatest frequency of noxious effects of radical relocation occur during the first month or two after such an event, it is important for interventions to be scheduled as soon as possible for maximum preventive potential. Medical social workers who plan nursing home placement should devote some efforts toward easing the stress experienced by patient and family. As other studies (Aldrich & Mendkoff, 1963; Kral et al., 1968; Markus et al., 1971; Miller & Lieberman, 1965; Lieberman, 1969) suggest, providers of long term care should design admission procedures, including careful follow-up, which will provide for maximum self-regulation and a minimum of psychological loss. If family, friends, and voluntary groups are encouraged to provide extra support perhaps before and certainly during the first few weeks after entry into a nursing home, the result might prevent unnecessary trauma and even deaths. The specific factors operative in the not-for-profit milieu which result in lowered entry-associated morbidity and mortality, could be identified and perhaps subsequently translated into policy and procedures to be adapted by proprietary homes. As it now stands, the reasons older patients are institutionalized supposedly involve their increased well being. Very few would choose to move to a nursing home because of a perceived improvement in life satisfaction. Yet this attempt to provide a better environment for care of their health may prove to be a morbid, if not fatal, event. Health care for the elderly is a much needed industry, but we must not allow the providing of it to be iatrogenic. It is time to devise ways and means to prevent unnecessary geriatric deaths due to institutionalization.

REFERENCES

Aldrich, C.K., & Mendkoff, E. Relocation of the aged and disabled: A mortality study. *Journal of the American Geriatrics Society*, 1963, *11*, 185–194.

Anderson, N., Holmberg, R.H., & Stone, L.B. *Nursing home care: Effects of ownership and administration*. Paper presented at the Gerontological Society meeting, St. Petersburg, November 8, 1967.

Barton, W.E. *Administration in Psychiatry*. Springfield, Illinois: Charles C. Thomas, 1962.

Bourestom, N., Pastalan, L., & Tars, S. *Forced relocation: Setting, staff and patients effects*. Final report of the Institute of Gerontology, University of Michigan, Ann Arbor, 1975.

Burgess, E.W. Social relations, activities, and personal adjustment. *American Journal Sociology*, 1954, *59*, 352–360.

Dobson, W.R., & Patterson, T.W. A behavioral evaluation of geriatric patients living in nursing homes as compared to a hospitalization group. *Gerontologist*, 1961, *1*, 135–139.

Donahue, W. Impact of living arrangements on ego development in the elderly. In *Pattern of living and housing of middle aged and older people* (PHS No. 1496). Washington, D.C.: U.S. Government Printing Office, 1965.

Epstein, L.J., & Simon, A. *Alternatives to state hospitalization for geriatric mentally ill.* Langley Porter Neuropsychiatric Clinics, San Francisco, 1967, dittoed paper.

Farrari, N. Freedom of choice. *Social Work,* 1963, *8,* 105–106.

Fried, M. Grieving for a lost home. In L.J. Duhl (Ed.), *The urban condition.* New York: Basic Books, 1963.

Friedsam, H.J. Reactions of older persons to disaster-caused losses: An hypothesis of relative deprivation. *Gerontologist,* 1961, *1,* 34–37

Goldfarb, A.I., Shahinian, S.P., & Turner, H. *Death rates of relocated nursing home residents.* Paper presented at the 17th annual meeting of the Gerontological Society, New York, 1966.

Huck, S. W., Cormier, W.H., & Bounds, W.G. *Reading statistics and research.* New York: Harper & Row, 1974.

Jasnau, K.F. Individualized versus mass transfer of nonpsychotic geriatric patients from mental hospitals to nursing homes, with special reference to the death rate. *Journal of the American Geriatrics Society,* 1967, *15,* 280–284.

Killian, E.C. Effects of geriatric transfers on mortality rates. *Social Work,* 1970, January, 19–26.

Kral, V.A., Grad, B., & Berenson, J. Stress reactions resulting from the relocation of an aged population. *Canadian Psychiatric Association Journal,* 1968, *13,* 201–209.

Lawton, M., & Yaffee, S. *Mortality, morbidity and voluntary change of residence.* Paper presented at the meeting of the American Psychological Association, Washington, September, 1967.

Levey, S., Kinloch, D., Stotsky, B., Ruchlin, H., & Oppenheim, W. *Nursing homes in Massachusetts: An analysis of costs and services.* New York: Department of Administrative Medicine, Mount Sinai School of Medicine, City University of New York, 1971.

Lieberman, M.A. The relationship of mortality rates to entering a home for the aged. *Geriatrics,* 1961, *16,* 515–519.

Lieberman, M.A., Prack, V.N., & Tobin, S.S. Psychological effects of institutionalization. *Journal of Gerontology,* 1968, *23,* 343–353.

Lieberman, M.A. Institutionalization of the aged: Effects of Behavior. *Journal of Gerontology,* 1969, *24,* 330–340.

Lieberman, M., Tobin, S., & Slover, D. *The effects of relocation on long-term geriatric patients.* Department of Health and Committee on Human Development, Chicago, 1971.

Markus, E., Blenker, M., Bloom., M., & Downs, T. The impact of relocation upon mortality rates of institutionalized aged persons. *Journal of Gerontology,* 1971, *26,* 537–541.

Markus, E., Blenker, M., Bloom, M. & Downs, T. Some factors and their association with past relocation mortality among institutionalized aged persons. *Journal of Gerontology,* 1972, *27,* 376–382.

Michelson, L.C. The new leisure class. *American Journal of Sociology,* 1954, *59,* 371–378.

Messer, M. Rate differences in selective attitude dimensions of the elderly. *Journal of Gerontology,* 1968, *8,* 245–249.

Miller, D., & Lieberman, M.A. The relationship of affect state adaptive reactions to stress. *Journal of Gerontology,* 1965, *20,* 492–497.

Ogren, E.H., & Linn, M.W. Male nursing home patients: Relocation and mortality. *Journal of the American Geriatrics Society,* 1971, *18,* 229–239.

Pegels, C.C. *Health Care and the Elderly.* Rockville, Maryland: Aspen Systems Corp., 1981.

Schoenberg, B., Carr, A., Peretz, D., & Kutscher, A.H. (Eds.). *Psychological management in medical practice.* New York: Columbia Univ. Press, 1970.

Schulz, R., & Aderman, D. Effect of residential change on the temporal distance to death of terminal cancer. *Omega: Journal of Death and Dying,* 1973, *4,* 157–162.

Sherwood, S. (Ed.). *Long-term care: A handbook for researchers, planners and providers.* New York: Spectrum Publications, 1975.

Sommer, K., & Ross, H. Social interaction on a geriatric ward. *International Journal of Social Psychiatry,* 1958, *4,* 128.

Stotsky, B.A. A controlled study of factors in a successful adjustment of mental patients to a nursing home. *American Journal of Psychiatry,* 1967, *123,* 1243–1251.

Stotsky, B.A. (ed.). *The nursing home and the aging psychiatric patient.* New York: Appleton-Century, 1970.

Turner, B., Tobin, S., & Lieberman, M.A. Personality traits as predictors of institutional adaptation among the aged. *Journal of Gerontology,* 1972, *27,* 61–68.

U.S. Congress, Senate, Special Committee on Aging. *Developments in aging, 1970.* Washington, D.C.: U.S. Government Printing Office, 1971.

An Alternative Health Delivery System for the Chronically Ill Elderly

Lawrence J. Weiss
Barbara W. Sklar

ABSTRACT. The present health care system is fragmented, uncoordinated, and too costly for the chronically ill, elderly patient. Project OPEN provides preventive health and social services in order to reduce costs and provide more effective care. This alternative delivery system is based on a consortium brokerage model which provides functional assessment, care plan development and service coordination. A randomized sample of 338 elderly individuals participated in a time series experiment. Client functional status, service utilization, and all health costs were collected for six months. The results indicated a maintenance in functioning levels, a decrease in acute hospitalizations, and a 20% reduction in health care costs for the demonstration participants as compared to the control group. Project OPEN provided more effective care while simultaneously reducing health expenditures to the chronically ill elderly.

One of the major problems and challenges of our health care delivery system is how to integrate long-term care services for the chronically ill and disabled elderly with the existing acute care system. Long-term care services are presently unavailable or inaccessible to the majority of the chronically ill elderly, except through the traditional methods of institutional care (acute hospital and skilled nursing facility). To access the traditional system of care, the chronically ill person generally reaches an acute or crisis stage before seeking treatment so that the services will be reimbursed. The pre-

Lawrence J. Weiss is Research Director of Project OPEN and Barbara W. Sklar is Project Director and Director of Geriatric Services, Mt. Zion Hospital and Medical Center in San Francisco.

This research was supported by the U.S. Department of Health and Human Services, Health Care Financing Administration (HCFA) Grant #95-P-97231/9. The findings reported here do not necessarily reflect policies of HCFA. Reprints may be requested from Lawrence J. Weiss, Mt. Zion Hospital and Medical Center, P.O. Box 7921, San Francisco, CA 94120.

83

sent study evaluates an alternative delivery system that emphasizes primary prevention or earlier intervention strategies for the chronically disabled elderly. This alternative system is not based on what is reimburseable, but on the promotion of health and social services in order to prevent further disease and disability.

The need for an alternative health care delivery system for the chronically ill elderly is evident by the demand placed on the existing system of health care by the ever increasing numbers and proportion of elderly within the population (Pegels, 1981), the incidence of chronic diseases with increasing age (National Center for Health Statistics, 1979; Somers, 1982), and rapidly increasing health expenditures (Fisher, 1980). Consequently, there has been a national response to the growing need for long-term care services. Community-based demonstration programs that provide alternative health and social maintenance, rehabilitative, and preventive services developed around the late 1970's. However, most demonstration programs have produced very little evidence to date as to their success or failure. A few long-term care demonstration programs have provided results indicating that they have enabled their participants to remain independent longer and have forestalled institutionalization (Quinn, 1982; Shoaf, 1980; Zawadski, 1982), have decreased the mortality rate (Skellie & Coan, 1980), and have decreased the costs of providing services (Lombardi, 1981; Shoaf, 1980). Unfortunately, many long-term care demonstration programs have not employed an experimental methodology. The present study reports on Project OPEN (Organizations Providing for Elderly Needs) at Mt. Zion Hospital and Medical Center in San Francisco. Project OPEN, through an experimental methodology, evaluated whether or not its demonstration participants received more effective care (as displayed by a maintenance or improvement in functional status over time) than a control group representing the existing system of care. The goals of the project were to prevent institutionalizations in acute hospitals and skilled nursing facilities and provide more cost-efficient care than the existing health care delivery system.

METHOD

The Project's research and evaluation methodology employed an experimental design, combining a randomized control group with a time series or pretest-multiple-posttest method. After the initial referral and randomization procedure, a baseline functional status assessment occurred at the participant's home and six months later (additional six-month intervals were not available to report at this time). A comparison of the initial baseline assessment scores and socio-demographics between the demonstration and control groups revealed very similar sample populations, verifying that the randomization process worked. All health and social service utilization and cost data were collected for each demonstration and control group participant for an approximate duration of 19 months.

Subjects

The sample was obtained from community referrals to Project OPEN. The selection criteria for the study consisted of any person 65 years of age or older who had Medicare A and B only (not Medicaid), resided within a certain urban geographic area, and had at least one chronic condition that made them at-risk of needing more dependent care, making it difficult to live or function independently. An example of an "at-risk" person was one who experienced a hospitalization within 30 days of being referred to the program or the loss of a spouse within the year. For the intake period, August 18, 1980 to March 31, 1982, Project OPEN enrolled 338 clients: 220 demonstration participants, 118 control participants. Of those persons who became active participants from the pool of referrals, 55% were referred to the program from an agency, 17% were self referrals, and the remaining 28% were referrals from family members, friends or physicians. No intervention occurred with the control group participants. They were, however, referred to other service programs if they were not willing to participate in the project.

The Project OPEN population mean age was 80 with the youngest participant being 66 years old, and the oldest participant being 99 years old. Seventy percent of the population were female. The ethnic distribution showed that 68% were white, 19% were Japanese, 11% were black, and 2% other. With regard to marital status, 45% were widowed, 30% were married, 14% were single and 11% were either separated or divorced. There were no economic criteria for admittance into the "Medicare only" program. As a result, 70% of the Project OPEN sample had annual incomes between $3,000 and $10,000. Twenty eight percent had some grammar school education, 48% had some high school and/or trade school, and 24% had college or graduate level education. Medically, 36% of participants had a primary diagnosis of cardiovascular disease. Most of the primary presenting problems at the time of referral were in the physical health domain (47%) and activities or instrumental activities of daily living (35%). Given the selection criteria and socio-demographics of the sample, the participants represented a middle and low-middle class chronically ill elderly population who were at-risk of needing more dependent levels of care, including institutionalization.

Procedure

A comprehensive functional assessment of each participants' needs was administered in an interview format by a trained professional in the subject's home. This structured interview solicited both the participant's perspective of their behavioral status and the professional's observations. A 6-month care plan was developed from the functional status assessment information by an interdisciplinary team of health professionals. A Project OPEN Service Coordinator (public health nurse or social worker) arranged for and monitored the service delivery, including the quantity and quality of services. The goal of service coordination was to provide continuous care based on an individual's level of functioning in order to keep the person as independent as possible. The project's extended Medicare services were comprehensive. The service package was designed to provide reimbursement for preventive and maintenance services which were better adapted for chronic illness and disability. The goal of the demonstration project was to provide quality care alternatives to unnecessary utilization of institutional care and simultaneously reduce health care expenditures. The study reported here compared the demonstration group participants who received the benefits of functional assessment, care plan development, service coordination, and extended Medicare services with the control group who did not receive the above process.

Measures

In order to test the research hypotheses and evaluate the program properly, two primary sets of data were collected: functional status and needs assessment; service utilization and costs.

Functional Status and Needs Assessment. The participants' level of functioning and assessment of service need was achieved through the comprehensive Functional Status Instrument (FSI), a modification of the "222" Patient Status Instrument developed by the 1975 National Center for Health Services Research Study on Adult Day Health Care and Home Care (Jones, McNitt, & McKnight, 1974). The FSI was designed to assess the chronically ill elderly person's functional status in the following seven areas: mental status or orientation, physical status, activities of daily living, instrumental activities of daily living, psychological status, social network, and environmental satisfaction. These seven FSI scales included already established instruments, some with slight modifications, and others with new or additional items.

The first FSI scale, mental status, adopted Kahn, Pollack, & Goldfarb's Mental Status Questionnaire (1961) and included items that the interviewer rated on judgement of orientation, communication of need, speech impairment, and behavior pattern. The range of scores for the mental status scale was 4 to 25, a higher score indicated lower functioning levels. (This applied to all FSI scale scores.) The second FSI scale was physical status. This scale included items on bed disability days, handling of medications, sight, hearing, foot care, dental care, and range of motion. The scores ranged from 7 to 55. The activities of daily living was the third FSI scale score (scores ranged from 11 to 68). This scale was a slight modification of Katz's (1963) Activities of Daily Living instrument. The fourth FSI scale adopted Lawton and Brody's (1969) Instrumental Activities of Daily Living (scores ranged from 12 to 50). Psychological status was the fifth FSI scale. This scale incorporated an abbreviated symptom checklist from Lowenthal and Associates' (1975) Psychosomatic Symptom Checklist, as well as items concerning decision making, life satisfaction, safety, and ability to manage one's own life. These FSI scale scores ranged from 4 to 31. The next FSI scale, social network, was developed for the present study. The items ranged from frequency and type of contact with family and friends, having a confidant, quality of helpers, to range and type of activities. The scores for the social network scale ranged from 19 to 94. The last FSI scale was environmental satisfaction. The items within this scale included building access, adequacy of living space, bathroom, meals, and laundry, and transportation satisfaction. Scores ranged from 7 to 14. The range of the sum of all scale scores possible was 64 to 337. A higher score indicated lower functioning levels.

During the development of the FSI, reliability was determined with a sample of 30 participants using three different methods: interviewer agreement at different times, test-retest agreement, and observer agreement. It was determined that the percent of exact agreement was 80%, 86%, and 92% respectively. The degree of internal consistency for each of the seven FSI scales as determined by the Alpha/Standard Item Alpha Reliability coefficient are reported in Table 1. The reliability coefficients indicated a fair amount of internal consistency among the items within the FSI scales. One additional psychometric technique was to validate the FSI scale scores. This was accomplished by comparing the actual FSI scale scores with the assessor's professional judgement rating of the participant's "level of functioning" on a 1 to 9 scale for overall functioning. Table 2 reports the Pearson correlation coefficients between the ratings and the FSI scale scores. The results clearly substantiated the validity of the FSI scales, except the social network scale which revealed a negatively significant correlation with the professional's overall rating of functional level. In sum, the FSI was reliable and

TABLE 1

Internal Consistency

of

FSI Scale Scores

SCALE	RELIABILITY COEFFICIENT (Alpha/Standard Item Alpha)
Mental Status/Orientation	.73
Physical Status	.32
Activities of Daily Living	.84
Instrumental Activities of Daily Living	.81
Psychological Status	.62
Social Network	.80
Environmental Satisfaction	.50

TABLE 2

Validity of FSI Scale Scores

Pearson Correlation Coefficient (r)

SCALE	Overall Rating (n=550)	Each Component Scale Rating (n=500)
Mental Status/Orientation	.36*	.56*
Physical Status	.33*	.34*
Activities of Daily Living	.56*	.61*
Instrumental Activities of Daily Living	.64*	.75*
Psychological Status	.25*	.38*
Social Network	-.24*	.10
Environmental Satisfaction	.27*	.29*

* = $p < .001$

valid enough to assess the functioning levels of the sample population.

Service utilization and costs. All the health and social services received by the participants, both demonstration and control, were monitored and documented within the database. The service utilization data included the type of service rendered, date of the service received, total number of units of service, and the actual cost of the service. The charges for each available service, ranging from meals, transportation, and senior center programs to professional and skilled nursing facility services, were established on a "unit of service" basis. Actual cost rates were determined and updated regularly. The project documented and compared all of the service charges for the duration of the program, regardless of source of payment. In order to accomplish this, internal documentation and billing mechanisms were established within the consortium and contracted agencies. The Explanation of Benefits (E.O.B.) was obtained from the third party payers (i.e., Blue Shield) to further substantiate any service utilization information collected.

RESULTS

The functional status initial hypothesis concerning participant functioning levels predicted that those in the demonstration group would maintain or improve their level of functioning over time, while the control group would decrease their level of functioning. Performing a standard t-test on the FSI scale data for the baseline and 6-month follow-up revealed that the demonstration group participants had one negative significant difference (activities of daily living scale), and one positive significant difference (environmental satisfaction scale). The control group, on the other hand, displayed significant t values in the predicted direction of a decrease in functioning over time on two scales and the total functioning score. The two scales were activities of daily living and the social network scale (Table 3). An analysis of variance (ANOVA) statistic on the total FSI scale score interaction between demonstration and control groups for baseline and 6-month follow-up assessments produced significant results $(F(1,80) = 8.46, p < .005)$, indicating that the Project OPEN process of health care delivery prevented or inhibited some deterioration in functioning levels.

Institutionalization

The second part of the first hypothesis predicted that the demonstration participants would have a lower rate of institutionalization, both acute hospitalizations and skilled nursing facility (SNF) placements, than the control group. The results for 19 months of data collection indicated that the percentage of demonstration clients ($n = 220$) admitted to an acute hospital was 29%, while the controls ($n = 118$) had a significantly higher rate of 41% (Critical Ratio (336) = 2.13, $p < .05$). During the same period of time, the SNF admission rate for the demonstration participants was 2.7% as com-

Table 3

Functional Status Instrument (FSI) Scale Scores

Scale	Demonstration				Control			
	n	Baseline Mean	6-Month Follow-up Mean	t	n	Baseline Mean	6-Month Follow-up Mean	t
Mental Status	165	4.85	4.82	-.22	53	5.33	5.52	-1.35
Physical Status	142	14.34	14.17	1.06	38	14.32	14.98	-.61
Activities of Daily Living(ADL)	159	17.83	18.51	-2.56**	51	17.42	18.34	-3.25**
Instrumental Activities of Daily Living(IADL)	137	22.36	22.71	-1.77	41	22.17	22.66	-1.35
Psychological	157	12.13	11.61	1.30	46	11.25	11.65	-1.43
Social Network	90	57.23	53.12	1.15	28	58.23	59.02	-2.22*
Environmental Satisfaction	159	8.32	8.01	3.17**	48	8.35	8.20	.84
TOTAL FSI SCALE SCORE	67	137.06	132.95	1.54	15	137.07	140.37	-2.29*

* $p < .05$ ** $p < .01$

91

pared to 6.8% for the control group. The difference was significant (Critical Ratio (336) = 1.67, $p < .05$, one-tailed). Clearly, Project OPEN demonstration participants utilized acute hospitals and SNF's significantly less than those who utilized the existing system. The acute hospital readmission rate was 39% for the demonstration group and 46% for the controls. The difference indicated a 7% higher rate for controls; this difference was not statistically significant. Once hospitalized, the demonstration participants stayed an average of 12.9 days, while the control group stayed an average of 15 days in the acute setting. This result was in the expected direction but not significant. However, the number of acute hospital days aggregated over the total sample produced a significantly smaller (t (336) = 2.64, $p < .01$) mean number of days for the demonstration group (6.05 days) than the control group (9.92 days). In short, a decrease in institutionalization resulted from a significant reduction in the acute hospital and SNF admission rates and total number of acute hospital days per capita. This reduction was not observed in the readmission rate or the length of stay.

Cost-Efficient Care

The second hypothesis predicted that the actual costs of all the medical, health, and social care provided to the demonstration clients within the alternate delivery system (including the cost of service coordination) would be equal to or less than the costs for the control group. The results indicated that after 19 months of data collection, the demonstration group participants (2790 client months) had a 20% reduction in total health care costs over the control group (1133 participant months). The average cost reduction was $175.78 per participant per month. The savings occurred primarily in the Medicare Part A or acute hospital services. Medicare Part A services accounted for 74% of the total costs for the control group and 56% of the demonstration group costs. The average total monthly cost per demonstration participant equaled $694 (including the cost of service coordination and other extended benefit services), while controls totalled $870. Separating these total costs, the extended benefit services which focused more on maintenance and preventive services (e.g., homemaker, transportation, appliances) rendered to demonstration participants averaged $193 per person per month, while the control group averaged $109. Medicare Part B or physician and outpatient services showed a high initial cost outlay for the demonstration participants but then tapered off, resulting in a lower average per month (demonstration = \$60 and control = \$95).

DISCUSSION

The results indicate that Project OPEN provides a more effective model of health care delivery for the chronically ill elderly than the present system. Through the OPEN process of functional assessment, service coordination, monitoring, and extending the benefit of in-home support services, the quality of patient care was improved, reductions in functional status were prevented, and, finally, institutional placements and overall costs were reduced. The results do not support previous cost findings of other long-term care demonstration projects which report add-on or increased costs (Quinn, 1982; Skellie, Mobley, & Coan, 1982). A partial explanation rests in the fact that Project OPEN focused more on prevention and earlier intervention by targeting a population of chronically ill elderly who were "at-risk" of needing more dependent services and not on a more dysfunctional, skilled nursing level population as did the other projects (Price, Ripps, & Piltz, 1980; Skellie, Mobley, & Coan, 1982; Zawadski, 1979). In addition, since Project OPEN participants were "Medicare only," they had more economic resources, achieved a higher educational level and had a different ethnic distribution than the other long-term care project populations. Project OPEN's positive outcome of maintaining functioning levels over time has been reported in other long-term care research projects (Lombardi, 1981; Quinn, 1982; Shoaf, 1980). Additional research is needed to compare in greater detail the differences in project findings and the substantive question of how targeting different levels of functioning prevents or inhibits further disability. Also, more longitudinal data is needed to substantiate the positive results that Project OPEN found after 6 months.

The changing population demographics, increased health care costs, service inadequacies and Project OPEN's research results underline the pressing need to develop an appropriate long-term care system responsive to the needs of the chronically ill elderly. A long-term care system should be a comprehensive, accessible, and coordinated network of health and social services. Unfortunately, federal and state policy today is built on a "tinker toy" structure of very weak connections, disorganization, overlapping jurisdiction, contradictory regulations and missing components (e.g., reimbursement for preventive and maintenance home care services). New public policy is needed, which would integrate into existing Medicare, Medicaid and other third party reimbursement mechanisms incentives for the provision of alternative health delivery systems which are community-based and provide services to the chronically ill elderly.

REFERENCES

Fisher, C.R. Differences by age groups in health care spending. *Health Care Financing Review*, 1980, *1*(4), 65-90.

Hicks, B., Raisz, H., Segal, J., & Doherty, N. The triage experiment in coordinated care for the elderly. *American Journal of Public Health*, 1981, *71*(9), 991-1003.

Jones, E.W., McNitt, B.J., & McKnight, E.M., *Patient classification for long term care* (DHEW Publication No. HRA 75-3107). Washington, D.C.: U.S. Government Printing Office, 1974.

Kahn, R.L., Pollack, M., & Goldfarb, A.I. Factors related to individual differences in mental status of institutionalized aged. In P. Hock & J. Zubin (Eds.), *Psychopathology of aging*. New York: Grune and Stratton, 1961.

Katz, S., Ford, A.B., Moskowitz, R.W., Jackson, B.A., & Jaffe, M.W. Studies of illness in the aged. The Index of ADL: A standardized measure of biological and psycho-social function. *Journal of the American Medical Association*, 1963, *185*, 914-919.

Lawton, M.P., & Brody, E.M. Assessment of older people: Self-maintaining and instrumental activities of daily living. *The Gerontologist*, 1969, *9*, 179-186.

Lombardi, T. *Nursing home without walls program.* Unpublished report, New York State Senate Health Committee, Room 612, Legislative Office Building, Albany, New York, August, 1981.

Lowenthal, M.F., Thurnher, M., Chiriboga, D., Beeson, D., Gigy, L., Lurie, E., Pierce, R., Spence, D., & Weiss, L. *Four stages of life: A comparative study of women and men facing transitions.* San Francisco: Jossey-Bass, 1975.

National Center for Health Statistics. *Current estimates from the health interview survey series 13, No. 130* (DHEW Pub. No. (PHS) 80-1551). Washington, D.C.: U.S. Government Printing Office, 1979.

Pegels, C.C. *Health care and the elderly.* Rockville, Maryland: Aspen, 1981.

Price, L.C., Ripps, H.M., & Piltz, D.M. *Third year evaluation of the Monroe county long term care program.* Unpublished report, Macro Systems, Inc., 8630 Fenton Street, Silver Spring, Maryland, 1980.

Quinn, J. *Triage II: Coordinated delivery of services to the elderly.* Unpublished executive summary report, 35 Apple Hill, Wethersfield, Connecticut, February, 1982.

Quinn, J., Segal, J., Raisz, H., & Johnson, C. (Eds.). *Coordinating community services for the elderly.* New York: Springer, 1982.

Shoaf, K. *Demonstration project report.* Unpublished report, Community Care Organization of Milwaukee County, Inc., 1845 North Farwell Ave. Suite 200, Milwaukee, Wisconsin, November, 1980.

Skellie, F.A., & Coan, R.E. Community-based long-term care and mortality: preliminary findings of Georgia's alternative health services project. *The Gerontologist*, 1980, *20*, 372-379.

Skellie, F.A., Mobley, G.M., & Coan, R.E. Cost-effectiveness of community-based long-term care: Current findings of Georgia's alternative health services project. *American Journal of Public Health*, 1982, *72*(4), 353-358.

Somers, A.R. Long-term care for the elderly and disabled: A new health priority. *The New England Journal of Medicine,* 1982, *307*(4), 221-226.

Weissert, W., Wan, T., Livieratos, B., & Katz, S. Effects and costs of day-care services for the chronically ill: A randomized experiment. *Medical Care,* 1980, *18*(6), 567-584.

Zawadski, R. *On-Lok senior health services: Toward a continuum of care.* Unpublished report, 1455 Bush Street, San Francisco, California, 1979; and personal communication, Summer, 1982.

Health, Prevention and Television: Images of the Elderly and Perceptions of Social Reality

Nancy Signorielli

ABSTRACT. This article examines the relationship between television, aging, health, and, to a lesser degree, prevention. It is based upon research conducted as part of Cultural Indicators, a 14 year research project examining trends in television content and viewer conceptions of social reality. The article focuses upon the presentation of older characters and old age in prime time network television drama, with special attention to what these images reveal about aging, health and prevention. The article also examines some viewer conceptions relating to these issues.

This research reveals that older people are a very small segment of the prime time network dramatic television character population. Moreover, characters of all ages, the elderly included, are generally healthy, slim, rarely wear glasses, and seem to eat "on the run." This research also shows that respondents who watch more television tend to believe that the elderly are a diminishing segment of our population. Those who watch a lot of television are also likely to exhibit views reflecting a general complacency about health and poor nutritional knowledge and behavior.

Aging, health, and prevention are processes that start with birth and continue throughout life. In regard to aging the different stages of the life cycle are roles that are learned from the numerous images about aging to which we are exposed during our lifetimes. Similarly, our knowledge about health and how to stay healthy also comes from many sources, some cultural. In fact, a recent report (U.S.

Requests for reprints may be sent to Nancy Signorielli, The Annenberg School of Communications, University of Pennsylvania, Philadelphia, PA 19104.

Dept. of Health, Education and Welfare, 1979) has called for a re-ordering of health priorities and noted that as much as half of U.S. mortality may be accounted for by culturally sustained behavioral and lifestyle factors. One of the most pervasive suppliers of such images, messages, and lessons is the world of television.

Television is the mainstream of our popular culture. It presents stable and vivid images of many different facets of life and society, including information about health and the life cycle. Television presents a common view of the world—one that enters the lives of practically all Americans for several hours each day. It enters the American home with little deviation or selectivity for an average of 30 hours each week; children and older folks watch somewhat more while teenagers watch somewhat less (Neilson, 1979). Television's entertainment programs and commercials, with their potential messages about health and aging, reach tens of millions of viewers, many of whom would not otherwise expose themselves to such information.

The world of television is, however, a world created primarily to serve the function of attracting viewers for commercials. It is a synthetic world in which every character, prop, theme, locale, action, and character is manufactured to attract the largest number of viewers at the least possible cost. The world of television is ruled by the principle of cost per thousand—how much money it costs to attract a thousand viewers. Moreover, not every viewer counts the same; the primary goal of prime time television is to attract viewers between 18 and 49—those in the prime earning and spending years of life.

The world of television may thus be thought of as a highly controlled assembly line product. Its people do not live or die but are created or destroyed to tell a story. The message of all stories emerges from the aggregate patterns of casting, characterization, and fate. Moreover, every dramatic program is structured to make its casting seem natural—but casting has a message all of its own.

Roles are created in direct relation to usefulness in the world of television. The most numerous are those for whom the world has more use—more jobs, adventure, sex, power, and other opportunities and life chances. These values are distributed as most resources are distributed—according to status and power. Dominant social groups tend to be over-represented and over-endowed, not only absolutely, but even in relation to their numbers in the real population. Minorities are defined as having less than their proportionate share of values and resources. In the world of television drama this means less usefulness and opportunities, and fewer and more stereotyped roles. Under-representation means restricted scope of action, stereotyped roles, diminished life chances, and undervaluation ranging from relative neglect to symbolic annihilation.

This does not mean to imply that faithful proportional representation of reality is necessarily fair or just. Artistic and dramatic functions require selection, amplification, and invention, all of which may deviate from what the census reports or what independent experience reflects. Reality provides a standard by which the nature and extent of the deviations can be measured. The important question is not so much whether there are deviations as what kind exist and with what consequences for thinking, action, and policy.

This paper will examine and discuss some of the things television tells us about age roles, especially what it means to be and/or become old. It will also look at the recurrent patterns of health information that are part of this inescapable mainstream of our widely shared symbolic environment. Finally, it will examine the relationship between television viewing and viewer conceptions relating to some of these issues. While some of the evidence is fragmentary and uneven, it nevertheless indicates the potential and promise of further work in this area.

THE ELDERLY ON TELEVISION: REVIEW OF PREVIOUS RESEARCH

The most pervasive finding of research on the image of the elderly on television has been their gross underrepresentation (see, for example, Rubin, 1982). In addition to underrepresentation, many studies have revealed that characterizations of the elderly are often misleading and inaccurate. Although the Grey Panther's "Media Watch" is not "academic" research, this group nevertheless provides useful information by monitoring the way senior citizens are presented on television. According to Lydia Braggar, chairperson of "Media Watch," old people are depicted as "ugly, toothless, sexless, incontinent, senile, confused and helpless. . .Old age has been so negatively stereotyped that is has become something to dread and feel threatened by" (O'Hallaren, 1977, p. 21). Similarly, Carmichael (1976, p. 128) has noted that the mass media presents older people as "slow, less intelligent, decrepit, sick, sex-less, ugly, and senile." A study by Peterson (1973) of 30 half-hour segments randomly sampled by day, time-slot, and network during one week of broadcasting on the other hand, revealed that the elderly were generally portrayed in proportion to their representation and that the image of the elderly was not entirely negative. She found that older people were portrayed as active (93 percent), independent (82 percent), and in good health (82 percent).

The underrepresentation of older people on television has been by far the most usual finding and noted by many researchers. Northcott (1975) analyzed evening (7–10 PM) dramatic programs with modern settings and found that characters over 64 accounted for only 7 out of 464 characters (1.5 percent). Moreover, five of these seven characters played minor roles. Greenberg (1980) and Greenberg, Simmons, Hogan, and Atkin (1980) found that characters over 65 made up only about 3 percent of the major characters in three yearly samples of prime-time network dramatic programming.

Over the past 14 years, as part of our Cultural Indicators project, my colleagues and I have examined the image of the elderly in week long samples of prime-time and weekend-daytime network television drama. This research revealed that from 1969 to 1978 characters over 65 made up only 2.3 percent of the prime-time population and only 1.4 percent of the weekend-daytime population (Gerbner, Gross, Signorielli, & Morgan, 1980).

Aronoff (1974) studied 2,741 major characters appearing in programs analyzed as part of the Cultural Indicators Project between 1969 and 1971. He found that the elderly comprised only 4.9 percent of the characters in non-cartoon network drama. Moreover, there were about the same number of elderly men and women. Aronoff also found that the chances of male villainy increased with age, as did their rate of failure. Older female characters failed more often than they succeeded. ''In a world of generally positive portrayals and happy endings, only 40 percent of older male and even fewer older female characters were presented as successful, happy, and good'' (p. 87).

Previous analyses of the Cultural Indicators data base have also focused upon aging. One study (Signorielli, 1974) revealed that the elderly made up only 5 percent of the sample of prime-time major characters in non-cartoon programs aired between 1969 and 1972. Another, more extensive, analysis of this data base (Signorielli, 1975) substantiated previous findings and revealed that age was one of three important dimensions of characterization: age was related to personality traits of characters in that young characters (especially children and adolescents) were usually portrayed with positive personality traits while older characters had more negative traits. This analysis also revealed that older males were usually presented as "ineffectual" and that older females were the most likely characters to be victims of violence.

Other findings about the way the elderly are presented on television often come from research whose main focus is not the elderly. For example, Downing's (1974) analysis of daytime serials revealed that female characters were younger than male characters and had a greater deterioration of occupational status as they grew older. Downing concluded that, "Still, the mature woman receives better representation in the daytime serial than on most other types of television programs" (p. 136).

METHODOLOGY

The research reported in this discussion was conducted as part of Cultural Indicators, an ongoing research project that has been examining trends in television content and conceptions of social reality since 1969 (Gerbner, Gross, Jackson-Beeck, Jeffries-Fox, & Signorielli, 1978; Gerbner, Gross, Signorielli, Morgan, & Jackson-Beeck, 1979; Gerbner, Gross, Morgan, & Signorielli, 1980a). The Cultural Indicators design consists of two inter-related procedures: (1) message system analysis—the annual content analysis of prime-time and weekend-daytime network television drama, and (2) cultivation analysis—determining the conceptions of social reality that television viewing tends to cultivate in different groups of viewers.

This study used data from annual content analyses that were generated by pairs of highly trained observers. These data isolate the gross, unambiguous, and commonly understood patterns of portrayal; they do not reflect what any particular individual viewer might see on any given evening, but rather what people, in general, are exposed to and absorb over long periods of time.

The entire sample was made up of twelve sample weeks that included all dramatic prime-time (8 to 11 PM EST) programs aired on ABC, CBS, and NBC during one week in the fall of each year from 1969 to 1979, plus three week-long samples from the spring of 1975, 1976 and 1981. Dramatic programs included television plays, movies shown on television, cartoons with a fictional story line, as well as situation comedies and crime-adventure shows. Variety programs, news and information, and sports programs broadcast during the sample week time parameters were not included. This twelve year (14 sample weeks) sample included 878 programs, 14,037 speaking characters, and 2,796 major characters (those who play roles essential to the story).

Each program in this sample was subjected to an extensive recording instrument that examined many different aspects of programming and characterization. (A complete description of this methodology, including reliability measures, may be found in Gerbner, Gross, Morgan, & Signorielli, 1980b). This analysis focused upon some of the data collected for major characters and, in certain instances, all speaking characters. The specific content items used in this analysis include category schemes for sex, race, character type ("good"-"bad"), success, role (comic-serious), committing violence, and victimization, and a number of items relating to health and well-being. Two age-related items were central to this analysis. Chronological age, an estimate of the actual age of the character, and social age, a functional category scheme used to characterize the life cycle as well as dramatic role. The categories included in the social age content item were: children/adolescents, young adults (typically the age between adolescence and more settled vocational and personal responsibilities), settled adults, and older adults (elderly).

Data from each sample week were subjected to an extensive reliability analysis to insure that the observations did not reflect instrument ambiguity or observer bias. Reliability was tested by having each content item in the instrument independently coded by two pairs of trained monitors. (To reflect a week's dramatic programming, the final data set consisted of a random selection from one of these two codings for each program.) An agreement coefficient was then calculated for each item.[1] Yearly coefficients ranged from .95 for sex to .66 for character type. The yearly coefficients for social age averaged .70.

---

[1]The assessment of reliability consists of the calculation of an agreement coefficient for each content item. Five computational formulae are used; their variations depend upon the scale type of the particular variable being analyzed. For the derivation of the formulae and a discussion of their properties see Krippendorff (1970, 1980). These coefficients range from +1.00 to −1.00 where +1.00 indicates perfect agreement and .00 is agreement due solely to chance. A coefficient of .50 indicates that performance is 50 percent above the level expected by chance. Acceptable levels of reliability are defined as follows: items with agreement coefficients of .8 or above are accepted unconditionally, items with coefficients between .6 and .8 are accepted conditionally, while items whose coefficients fall between .5 and .6 are used with extreme caution. All items used in this analysis meet these standards.

THE ELDERLY ON TELEVISION:
RESULTS OF CURRENT RESEARCH

Age is a strong determinant of who appears most and gains most on television. Table 1 shows the age distribution in real life and in the world of prime-time network dramatic television. In contrast to the distribution of age groups in the American population, the television curve bulges in the middle years and grossly underrepresents both younger and older people. More than half of television's dramatic population is between 25 and 45. Individuals under 19, who number about a third of the U.S. population, make up only a tenth of the fictional population. Those over 65, comprising about 11 percent of the U.S. population, make up only 2.3 percent of the fictional world. Rather strikingly, this pattern of over and underrepresentation seems to reflect the profile of expendable consumer income by age. Television is thus populated by those to whom its programs, and especially its commercials, are pitched—the group the industry would call the "prime demographic market."

In the world of prime-time drama men outnumber women by

Table 1

Comparison of the Age Distribution
of TV Characters with the 1980 U.S. Census
(1969-1981)

	U.S.	Prime-Time	
	%	N	%
Under 5 years	7.2	31	0.2
From 5-9 years	7.4	205	1.5
From 10-14 years	8.1	436	3.2
From 15-19 years	9.3	639	4.7
From 20-24 years	9.4	970	7.1
From 25-29 years	8.6	1886	13.8
From 30-34 years	7.8	1866	13.6
From 35-39 years	6.2	2119	15.5
From 40-44 years	5.2	1706	12.5
From 45-49 years	4.9	1521	11.1
From 50-54 years	5.2	1069	7.8
From 55-59 years	5.1	568	4.1
From 60-64 years	4.5	374	2.7
From 65-69 years	3.9	186	1.4
From 70-74 years	3.0	83	0.6
From 75-79 years	2.1	20	0.1
From 80-84 years	1.3	9	0.1
85 years and over	1.0	12	0.1
Total	100.0	13700	100.0

three to one. This finding has profound consequences for all that happens in that world. While women actually outnumber men among characters in their early twenties, as they grow older their numbers fall to four or five times below the number of men and their usefulness declines.

Table 2 gives the percent of men and women in each age group in the U.S. and on television. In prime time, the age distribution of women, compared to that of men, favors women under 30. While women are most concentrated in the 20 to 29 age group, men are most concentrated in the 30 to 40 age bracket. The distribution of age roles by race, as well as gender (Table 2) also reveals the value structure of the symbolic world. Again, the age distributions of both white and non-white men and women bulge in the middle. But, while white men dominate the age of dramatic authority between 35 and 50, non-white men are concentrated between 25 and 40. Non-white men age like women, especially white women, rather than like white men. Finally, non-white women age even slower than their white counterparts—about half of all non-white women are between 20 and 34.

Nevertheless, even though women on television are younger than men, among major characters women "age" much faster. As women age, they are cast in roles with fewer romantic possibilities. A comparison of the chronological age and social (role related) age of prime-time major characters reveals that as early as the teen years, the percentage of female characters (45.2 percent) assigned to the older social and dramatic category of young adult is greater than the percentage of males of the same age (36.7 percent) assigned to such roles. In their twenties, only 28.2 percent of the men, but 36.9 percent of the women are cast as settled adults (the rest, of course, are young adults). Among characters between 50 and 64, 11.3 percent of the men and 14.7 percent of the women are cast as old characters. Among characters 65 and older, 23.3 percent of the men still play settled adult roles and 76.7 percent are cast as old, but over 90 percent of the women of the same chronological age are cast as old.

We thus find that the character population is structured to provide a relative abundance of younger women for older men, but no such abundance of younger men is found for older women. Men age slower and enjoy life longer. Television perpetuates an inequitable and unfair, if conventional, pattern.

Characterizations of major characters in prime-time drama also vary according to social age roles. In Table 3 we find that the eval-

Table 2

Age Distribution of Male and Female, White and Other Race
Characters on Prime-Time Network Drama
(1969-1981)

	All Men		White Men		Non-White Men	
	U.S.	Prime Time	U.S.	Prime Time	U.S.	Prime Time
N =		9908		8724		1172
	%	%	%	%	%	%
Under 5 years	7.6	0.1	7.1	0.1	10.2	0.5
From 5-9 years	7.8	1.3	7.3	1.2	10.1	2.2
From 10-14 years	8.5	2.8	8.1	2.3	10.4	6.0
From 15-19 years	9.8	3.9	9.4	3.5	11.5	7.0
From 20-24 years	9.7	4.8	9.5	4.6	10.8	5.7
From 25-29 years	8.8	11.1	8.7	10.5	9.3	15.6
From 30-34 years	7.9	13.7	8.0	13.0	7.5	18.9
From 35-39 years	6.2	16.9	6.4	16.9	5.6	16.8
From 40-44 years	5.2	14.2	5.3	14.8	4.7	9.8
From 45-49 years	4.9	12.8	5.1	13.3	4.1	8.4
From 50-54 years	5.1	9.0	5.4	9.6	3.8	3.9
From 55-59 years	5.0	4.5	5.3	4.9	3.4	1.5
From 60-64 years	4.2	2.9	4.6	3.1	2.7	1.4
From 65-69 years	3.5	1.3	3.8	1.3	2.3	1.0
From 70-74 years	2.6	0.6	2.8	0.6	1.6	0.9
From 75-79 years	1.7	0.1	1.8	0.1	1.1	0.3
From 80-84 years	0.9	0.0	1.0	0.0	0.5	0.0
85 years and over	0.6	0.1	0.7	0.1	0.4	0.1

	All Women		White Women		Non-White Women	
	U.S.	Prime Time	U.S.	Prime Time	U.S.	Prime Time
N =		3783		3380		396
	%	%	%	%	%	%
Under 5 years	6.9	0.3	6.4	0.3	9.3	0.0
From 5-9 years	7.0	2.1	6.6	1.9	9.2	3.3
From 10-14 years	7.7	4.1	7.3	4.1	9.5	4.3
From 15-19 years	8.9	6.7	8.6	6.7	10.5	6.6
From 20-24 years	9.1	13.2	8.9	13.2	10.3	12.9
From 25-29 years	8.4	20.7	8.3	20.6	9.3	21.7
From 30-34 years	7.6	13.5	7.6	13.3	7.8	15.2
From 35-39 years	6.1	11.9	6.1	12.1	5.9	9.6
From 40-44 years	5.1	8.0	5.1	8.0	5.0	7.6
From 45-49 years	4.9	6.8	5.0	6.7	4.5	7.1
From 50-54 years	5.2	4.8	5.4	4.9	4.3	4.5
From 55-59 years	5.3	3.3	5.6	3.3	3.8	3.0
From 60-64 years	4.7	2.3	5.0	2.4	3.1	1.8
From 65-69 years	4.2	1.5	4.5	1.4	2.8	2.0
From 70-74 years	3.4	0.6	3.7	0.6	2.0	0.5
From 75-79 years	2.5	0.2	2.8	0.2	1.4	0.0
From 80-84 years	1.6	0.1	1.8	0.1	0.8	0.0
85 years and over	1.3	0.0	1.5	0.0	0.6	0.0

Table 3

Evaluation of Major Characters
on Prime-Time Network Drama
(1969-1981)

	Children and Adolescents		Young Adults		Settled Adults		Older Adults		Total	
	Men	Women	Men	Women	Men	Women	Men	Women	Men	Women
N =	112	53	370	228	1382	495	70	23	1979	814
	%	%	%	%	%	%	%	%	%	%
Character Type										
"Good"	57.1	52.8	57.8	60.5	55.8	61.8	44.3	47.8	55.7	60.6
Mixed	38.4	39.6	28.9	32.9	28.5	31.9	38.6	43.5	29.7	33.0
"Bad"	4.5	7.5	13.2	6.6	15.7	6.1	17.1	8.7	14.6	6.3
Success										
Successful	38.4	35.8	37.3	39.0	41.0	43.2	37.1	17.4	39.8	40.9
Mixed	49.1	50.9	43.0	46.5	39.0	44.0	40.0	47.8	40.7	45.1
Unsuccessful	12.5	13.2	19.7	14.5	19.9	12.5	22.9	34.8	19.4	13.9
Role										
Light/Comic	14.3	9.4	17.0	19.7	13.2	17.4	24.3	13.0	14.5	60.6
Mixed	28.6	43.4	24.3	23.7	17.6	25.9	22.9	39.1	19.8	33.0
Serious	57.1	47.2	58.6	56.6	69.2	56.8	52.9	47.8	65.8	6.3

uation of major characters as "good" or "bad" is related to these roles: as men age, proportionately more are portrayed as "bad." For females, more young girls and older women are portrayed as "bad" than are young or middle-aged women. An obvious and important difference is that proportionately fewer older characters are "good."

Age-related chances for success are also presented in Table 3. The percent of men in each age role who are successful is about the same. As women age, however, the percent who are successful is similar for girls, young and middle-aged women, but drops to 17 percent for older women. In fact, more older women are unsuccessful than are successful—something not seen for any other group. Casting a character in a comic, serious, or mixed role is also related to age. As Table 3 shows, among major characters, the elderly, especially elderly men, are less likely to portray serious roles than are characters in the younger age-roles. Moreover, older men are much more likely than younger men to be cast in a comic role.

On television, older characters, especially older women are more likely to be portrayed as formerly married or widowed (36.4 percent) than married (27.3 percent). They are also quite likely to have children (54.5 percent as compared to 32.3 percent of middle-aged women) but are considerably less likely to be involved in a romantic relationship. Only 9.1 percent of older women as compared to 59.6 percent of young women and 50.2 percent of middle-aged women are portrayed as being involved in a romantic relationship. Older men are also more likely to be portrayed as formerly married or widowed (39.3 percent) than married (17.9 percent). Moreover, on television, men are less likely than women to have children (35.7 percent of older men and 21.9 percent of middle-aged men have children) and a little less likely to be involved romantically (10.7 percent of older men, 34.7 percent of middle-aged men, and 40.2 percent of young men are involved in romantic relationships).

As is true of women of all ages, a large percentage of older women are presented as not working—29 percent are unemployed, 14 percent could not be coded (no information given) on this item, and 14 percent retired. While young and middle-aged men are usually shown working (only 17 percent of the young men and 8 percent of the middle-aged men could not be coded on occupation), older men are presented somewhat differently—only 9 percent could not be coded on occupation, 7 percent were unemployed, and 20 percent were retired. Less than 1 percent of the middle-aged men were retired.

The world of television is one that is dominated by violence and while characters of all ages are likely to take part in the violence (see Table 4), the patterns of involvement for older characters are somewhat different from those of younger characters. Among adult major characters, older men and especially old women are less likely to be involved in violence, but when involved, old men are the only group who are more likely to commit violence than be a victim of it (they are 1.14 times as likely to hurt others than be hurt) and old women are six times as likely to be hurt or killed than to hurt or kill others. Examination of who kills or is killed reveals that old men, like men of all ages, are more likely to kill than be killed; old women, however, are *only* the victims of lethal violence—they never kill anyone else.

HEALTH ON TELEVISION:
PATTERNS OF PORTRAYAL

Despite all the mayhem, the characters on television rarely are in need of medical help. Table 5 reveals that characters of all ages are seldom physically ill; overall, only 8 percent are so categorized. Even older characters exhibit less physical illness than one would expect; only 10 percent of the older men and 13 percent of the older

Table 4

Committing Violence and Victimization
of Major Characters
on Prime-Time Network Drama
(1969-1981)

	Children Adolescents		Young Adults		Settled Adults		Older Adults		Total	
	Men	Women	Men	Women	Men	Women	Men	Women	Men	Women
N =	112	53	370	228	1382	495	70	23	1979	814
	%	%	%	%	%	%	%	%	%	%
Violence By	27.7	20.8	50.8	28.1	47.5	25.7	34.3	4.3	46.8	25.8
Victimized	42.0	24.8	56.5	43.0	49.9	26.3	30.0	26.1	50.5	26.1
Involved In Violence	46.4	35.8	63.2	48.7	59.8	36.2	45.7	26.1	59.6	40.0
Violence-Victim Ratio	-1.52	-1.18	-1.11	-1.53	-1.05	-1.02	+1.14	-6.00	-1.08	-1.22
	%	%	%	%	%	%	%	%	%	%
Killer	2.7	1.9	13.2	3.9	11.7	3.6	8.6	0.0	11.6	3.4
Killed	0.9	1.9	5.9	2.2	5.4	2.2	5.7	13.0	5.5	2.6
Involved In Killing	3.6	1.9	15.9	6.1	14.3	5.3	12.9	13.0	14.2	5.5
Killer-Killed Ratio	+3.00	+1.00	+2.23	+1.8	+2.16	+1.64	+1.5	-0.0	+2.12	+1.33

Risk ratios are obtained by dividing the more numerous of these two roles
by the less numerous within each group. A plus sign indicates that there
are more violents or killers than victims or killed and a minus sign
indicates that there are more victims or killed than violents or killers.
A ratio of 0.00 means that there were no victims or killers or violents
or killed. A +0.00 ratio means that there were some violents or killers
but no victims or killed; a -0.00 ratio means there were victims or killed
but no violents or killers.

women are seen as having an illness that requires some medically-
related treatment. Nevertheless, doctors and nurses abound on these
programs. The typical viewer of prime time programs sees about 12
doctors and 6 nurses each week, including 3 doctors and 1 nurse in
major roles. Very few characters are mentally ill or physical handicapped. Moreover, characters, including the elderly, almost always

are ambulatory and rarely have sight impairments; only one in five older men and one in four older women have sight impairments.

While smoking does not occur very often on television, Table 5 shows that older characters smoke somewhat more than younger characters—14 percent of the older men and 1 in 5 older women smoke. On the other hand, social drinking of alcoholic beverages abounds. Adult television characters, especially the settled adults,

Table 5

Health and Health-Related Behaviors
of Major Characters
on Prime-Time Network Drama
(1969-1981)

	Children and Adolescents		Young Adults		Settled Adults		Older Adults		Total	
	Men	Women	Men	Women	Men	Women	Men	Women	Men	Women
N =	112	53	370	228	1382	495	70	23	1979	884
	%	%	%	%	%	%	%	%	%	%
Handicapped	3.6	1.9	2.7	1.3	2.2	1.0	4.3	4.3	2.4	1.4
Physical Illness	9.8	9.4	9.2	7.9	7.3	7.3	10.0	13.0	7.9	8.2
Mental Illness	2.7	1.9	5.7	3.9	2.6	1.0	2.9	0.0	3.3	2.0
N =	28	14	67	54	303	132	14	5	426	211
	%	%	%	%	%	%	%	%	%	%
Smokes	0.0	0.0	6.0	3.7	12.2	2.3	14.3	20.0	10.8	2.8
Drinks	7.1	0.0	20.9	24.1	42.2	45.5	35.7	20.0	35.9	35.5
Alcoholic	0.0	0.0	0.0	0.0	2.0	0.0	7.1	20.0	1.6	0.5
Restricted Mobility	3.6	0.0	4.5	0.0	1.0	0.0	0.0	0.0	1.6	0.0
N =	16	7	48	36	220	90	11	4	306	140
	%	%	%	%	%	%	%	%	%	%
Sight Impairment	12.6	0.0	2.1	0.0	9.6	7.8	18.2	25.0	9.2	6.4

are quite likely to be seen having a drink, although very few are shown as alcoholics. Interestingly, proportionately more older characters than those in any other age group are portrayed as alcoholics.

In regard to nutrition on prime-time television, a pilot study (Gerbner, Morgan, & Signorielli, 1982) conducted on a week-long sample of prime-time dramatic programming broadcast in 1978, revealed that eating and/or drinking occur about 10 times each hour. Three-quarters of all dramatic characters, or some 15 each night, eat, drink, or talk about it, often more than once. Prime-time nutrition, however, is anything but balanced or relaxed: grabbing a snack (39 percent of all eating-drinking episodes) is virtually as frequent as breakfast, lunch, and dinner combined (42 percent). In episodes involving drinking, the most prevalent beverages are alcoholic. Coffee and tea are next. When eating and drinking occur simultaneously, more than half of the episodes are a meal with coffee, tea, or alcohol.

This pilot study also revealed that obesity, a problem than plagues from 25 to 45 percent of the American population, depending on the estimate, claims few victims on television. We found fewer than 6 percent of all males and 2 percent of all females (none of them leading characters) obese. Elderly characters and minorities were a little more likely to be presented as somewhat overweight, but it must be stressed that, overall, very few characters in any age or racial group were overweight.

An analysis of commercials (Gerbner, Gross, Morgan, & Signorielli, 1981) on prime-time and weekend-daytime programs revealed that food advertising accounts for more than a quarter of these commercials. Furthermore food related activities (including mention of food or drink) occurred in over 40 percent of them. Sweets, snacks, and non-nutritious ("junk") foods made up nearly half of food commercials; nutritional appeals were noted in only 9 percent and stressed in another 7 percent of food commercials.

AGING AND HEALTH ON TELEVISION: SUMMARY OF CONTENT FINDINGS

Overall, the most prevalent image of the older adult on television is one of invisibility; their small numbers and considerable underrepresentation greatly restrict the types of roles in which they will be seen. Older men and women are also presented quite differently.

Men, with their greater propensity to commit violence (and less likelihood to be victimized), emerge as considerably more powerful than women. Older women are presented in an especially negative way in that they are the only group who are more likely to be unsuccessful than successful and, when involved in violence, are much more likely to be hurt than to hurt others.

In regard to health issues, although the basic image is one of generally healthy people, older characters are a little more likely to be ill than younger characters. Also, in areas reflecting health-related habits (smoking, drinking, and weight), older people are presented in a less favorable light—they are the group who are most likely to be alcoholics, smokers, and a little more likely to be overweight.

VIEWER CONCEPTIONS OF AGING AND HEALTH

Isolating the image of older people and health-related practices on television is just one part of the story. How do these images affect viewers—what are the lessons viewers derive from television about growing old and being old in our society? What are the health implications of exposure to these messages embedded in our daily television fare? These are the questions our cultivation analyses attempt to answer.

Cultivation analysis is the investigation of the consequences of television's ongoing and pervasive system of cultural messages. Since it is based upon the premise that television's images cultivate the dominant tendencies of our culture's beliefs, ideologies, and world views, the observable independent contributions can only be relatively small. But just as an average temperature shift of a few degrees can lead to an ice age or the outcomes of elections can be determined by slight margins, so too can a relatively small but pervasive influence make a crucial difference. The "size" of an "effect" is far less critical than the direction of its steady contribution.

My colleagues and I have found that amount of exposure to television is an important indicator of the strength of its contributions to ways of thinking and acting. For heavy viewers, television virtually monopolizes and subsumes other sources of information, ideas, and consciousness. Thus, we have suggested that the more time one spends "living" in the world of television, the more one likely one is to report perceptions of social reality which can be traced to (or are congruent with) television's most persistent representations of life and society. Accordingly, we have examined the difference that amount of viewing makes in people's images, expectations, assumptions and behaviors (Gerbner, Gross, Morgan, & Signorielli, 1980a, 1982; Gerbner, Gross, Signorielli, Morgan, & Jackson-Beeck, 1979; Gerbner, Gross, Jackson-Beeck, Jeffries-Fox, & Signorielli. 1978).

Some answers to the first question (conceptions about aging) posed above come from a cultivation analysis of data from the National Council on Aging's "Myth and Reality of Aging" survey conducted by Louis Harris and Associates in 1974 (Gerbner, Gross, Signorielli, & Morgan, 1980). We constructed an index from the responses to statements asserting the number, the health, and the longevity of older people are declining.[2] A high score on this index reflects a generalized belief that old people represent a diminishing rather than growing segment of American society.

This analysis revealed a significant positive relationship between amount of television viewing and scores on this index. The more people, especially young people, watch television, the more they tend to perceive old people in generally negative and unfavorable terms. Heavy viewers believe significantly more than light viewers that old people are a vanishing breed. The correlation of .10 ($p < .001$; $N = 3772$) is not reduced by controls for education, income, sex, or age and it is much stronger for younger people; the correlation is .20 ($N = 1076$) for those under thirty.

Another analysis of a question in the National Council on Aging survey relating to the mobility of both the respondent and older people also sheds some light about viewer perceptions of aging. As noted above, the general image of the elderly on television is one of basically good health—very few older characters are physically or mentally ill, few have sight impairments, and even fewer have any problems with mobility.

Respondents were asked whether "walking or climbing stairs" was a very or somewhat serious problem for themselves and also for most people over 65. The first question (is mobility a problem for you?) showed a significant relationship, controlling for sex, age, education, race, income, and newspaper reading, between television viewing and responding that the respondent's mobility was a

---

[2]Factor analysis revealed that these three statements measured a single dimension. The variables produce a moderate but acceptable alpha of .56 and more than adequately pass a series of validity checks (Gonzalez, 1979).

very or somewhat serious problem ($r = .08$ $P < .001$; $N = 3174$). This finding is not surprising in that those who are more likely to have these problems probably spend more time at home and are thus more likely to watch more television.[3]

However, given that respondents' perceptions of the problems those over 65 have walking and climbing stairs may be influenced by the state of their own mobility, the analysis used the assessment of the respondent's mobility as a control. This analysis revealed that for those respondents whose *own* mobility was problematic there was a significant *negative* relationship between television viewing and responding that the mobility of those over 65 was a very or somewhat serious problem. That is, those who described themselves as having problems walking or climbing stairs, when they watched more television did not think that those over 65 had similar problems. This negative relationship also held up under controls for sex, age, education, race, income, and newspaper reading ($r = -.16$, $p < .001$; $N = 623$). There was no relationship between television viewing and perceptions of the problems people over 65 have walking or climbing stairs for those respondents who did not have mobility problems. It may be that those who have problems walking or climbing stairs are much more sensitive to these issues and when watching television are more sensitive to how these issues are presented.

We thus find that while the invisibility of the older person on television serves to cultivate in viewers a sense that being old is negative (respondents believe that the elderly do not really exist and that people, especially women, get old rather early in life), television does not cultivate only inaccurate or negative images. Rather, respondents who have problems walking and climbing stairs do not believe that mobility is a serious or very serious problem for most people over 65.

In regard to the second question, information about prevention and the health implications of exposure to television messages is scarce. We know that television tends to monopolize the cultural participation of the less educated, lower income groups. A study

---

[3]Data from other analyses also reveals that television viewing is also related to smoking and drinking. Analysis of data in the 1977 and 1978 NORC General Social Surveys revealed that non-smokers averaged 2.65 hours of viewing a day while cigarette smokers average 3.01 hours of television each day. Television viewing is, however, negatively associated with drinking alcoholic beverages for respondents who are white, between 18 and 19, college educated, or in excellent health (Gerbner, Morgan, & Signorielli, 1982).

conducted by General Mills (1979) shows that these groups have the poorest health and nutritional opportunities and are the most in need of valid information about health. This study also found that, next to doctors, television was the most frequently cited source of health information and that those who did choose television (vs. those who did not) manifested a distinct profile (Gerbner, Morgan, & Signorielli, 1982). In most demographic groups (defined by sex, social class, and place of residence), those who chose television programs as a source of information about health were significantly more likely to be categorized as "complacent" (vs. "concerned") on health attitudes; as holding "old" (vs. "new") health values; as being a "non-exerciser" on physical fitness; and as being "poorly-informed" (vs. "well" or "somewhat-informed") in terms of health information.

These data cannot support the argument that television contributes to poor health routines and a lack of awareness of health information (although they are consistent with such a notion). But they do suggest that those who credit television as a main source of information, even with other things held constant, are not among the more health-minded segments of the population.

Data from a 1979 study conducted by the Roper Organization for Virginia Slims (Gerbner, Morgan, & Signorielli, 1982) reveals that those who watch more television, other things held constant, are more likely to be complacent about eating, drinking, and exercise. While this association holds up within most subgroups, there are interesting exceptions which may be explained by a process my colleagues and I call "mainstreaming" (Gerbner, Gross, Morgan, & Signorielli, 1980a).

The "mainstream" can be thought of as a relative commonality of outlooks that television tends to cultivate. "Mainstreaming" means the sharing of that commonality among heavy viewers in those demographic groups whose light viewers hold divergent views. In other words, differences deriving from other factors and social forces may be diminished or even absent among heavy viewers. Thus, in some cases we should only find evidence for cultivation within those groups who are "out" of the mainstream. In other cases, we may find that viewing "moderates" attitudes in groups whose light viewers tend to hold extreme views. That is, groups who share a relative commonality of outlooks cultivated by television (the "mainstream" view) will often show weak or no association between amount of viewing and a given perspective, while strong relationships may be found for those groups whose lighter viewers do *not* share that outlook. Thus, cultivation may often imply a convergence into a more homogeneous "mainstream," rather than absolute, across-the-board increments.

For example, in regard to diet and nutrition, a "mainstreaming" pattern is evident for different age groups. There is virtually no relationship between amount of viewing and being unconcerned about diet and nutrition for older people: older people are more likely to be unconcerned regardless of viewing; they are already "in" the "mainstream." Younger and middle-aged respondents, on the other hand, show evidence of the cultivation of nutritional complacency. For respondents between 18 and 29 the relationship between television viewing and nutritional complacency as measured by gamma is .17 ($p < .001$; $N = 1085$) and for respondents between 30 and 49 gamma is .18 ($p < .001$; $N = 1203$). The farther away from the mainstream, the stronger the cultivation.

CONCLUSION

Television viewing is deeply integrated into different styles of life, with powerful implications for health practices. A variety of findings, though preliminary and often indirect, lend credence to the notion that television may have a considerable impact upon the public's images, knowledge, and behaviors. Television programs are a frequently cited source of health information; those who choose them, and/or heavier viewers, seem relatively neglectful and complacent about their physical well-being, are less informed about health, and exercise less. Heavy viewing also goes with getting less satisfaction from one's health and high confidence in the medical community. In addition, the very act of watching television may generate behaviors and habits with clear health implications in the areas of smoking, eating, and drinking.

With regard to health related program and commercial content, the portrayals of illness, doctors, nutrition, obesity, driving safety, smoking, and drinking reveal a serious conflict with realistic guidelines for health and medicine. Research on the contributions of these portrayals to specific conceptions of health and medicine is scarce. But the pattern of findings indicates that television viewing is associated with a convergence of the heavier viewers upon paradoxical and disjointed "mainstream" conceptions and practices.

The cultivation of ignorance and neglect, especially among otherwise relatively enlightened viewers, coupled with an unrealistic belief in the magic of medicine, is likely to perpetuate unhealthy lifestyles, hurt patients and health professionals, and frustrate efforts at health education. If culturally sustained health hazards are the new frontier in health promotion and disease prevention, there is a need for greater mobilization of effort and resources in a central sector of that frontier. The first step toward such mobilization is the fuller, broader, and more sustained study of the messages television conveys about health and a refinement of their contributions to the health conceptions and behaviors of various groups of viewers.

REFERENCES

Arnoff, C. Old age in prime time. *Journal of Communication,* 1974, *24*(4), 86-87.

Carmichael, C.W. Communication and gerontology: Interfacing disciplines. *Journal of the Western Communication Association,* 1976, *40,* 121-129.

Downing, M. Heroine of the daytime serial. *Journal of Communication,* 1974, *24*(2), 130-137.

General Mills, Inc. *The General Mills American family report, 1978-79: Family health in an era of stress.* Minneapolis: General Mills, 1979.

Gerbner, G., Gross, L., Jackson-Beeck, M., Jeffries-Fox, S., & Signorielli. N. Cultural indicators: Violence profile no. 9. *Journal of Communication,* 1978, *28*(3), 176-207.

Gerbner, G., Gross, L., Morgan, M., & Signorielli, N. The mainstreaming of America: Violence profile no. 11. *Journal of Communication,* 1980, *30*(3), 10-29. (a)

Gerbner, G., Gross, L., Morgan, M., & Signorielli, N. Violence profile no. 11: Trends in network television drama and conceptions of social reality. The Annenberg School of Communications, University of Pennsylvania, 1980. (b)

Gerbner, G., Gross, L., Morgan, M., & Signorielli, N. *Aging with television commercials: Images on television commercials and dramatic programming, 1977-1979.* The Annenberg School of Communications, University of Pennsylvania, 1981.

Gerbner, G., Gross, L., Morgan, M., & Signorielli, N. Charting the mainstream: Television's contributions to political orientations. *Journal of Communication,* 1982, *32*(2), 100-127.

Gerbner, G., Gross, L., Signorielli, N., & Morgan M. Aging with television: Images on television drama and conceptions of social reality. *Journal of Communication,* 1980, *30*(1), 37-47.

Gerbner, G., Gross, L., Signorielli, N., Morgan, M., & Jackson-Beeck, M. The demonstration of power: Violence profile no. 10. *Journal of Communication,* 1979, *24*(3), 177-196.

Gerbner, G., Morgan, M., & Signorielli, N. Programming health portrayals: What viewers see, say, and do. *Television and behavior: ten years of scientific progress and implications for the eighties (Vol 2): Technical reviews.* Washington D.C.: U.S. Government Printing Office, 1982.

Gerbner, G., & Signorielli, N. *Women and minorities in television drama: 1969-1978.* The Annenberg School of Communications, University of Pennsylvania, 1979.

Gonzalez, M. Television and people's images of old age. Masters thesis, University of Pennsylvania, 1979.

Greenberg, B.S. *Life on television.* Norwood, New Jersey: Ablex Publishing, 1980.

Greenberg, B.S., Simmons, K.W., Hogan, L., & Atkin, C. Three seasons of television characters: A demographic analysis. *Journal of Broadcasting,* 1980, *24*(1) 49-60.

Krippendorff, K. Bivariate agreement coefficients for the reliability of data. In E.F. Borgatta (Ed.), *Sociological methodology: 1970.* San Francisco: Jossey-Bass, 1970.

Krippendorff, K. *Content analysis: An introduction to its methodology,* Beverly Hills: Sage Publications, 1980.

Neilson report on television. Northbrook, Ill.: A.C. Nielson, 1979.

Northcott, H. Too young, too old: Age in the world of television. *The Gerontologist,* 1975, *15*(2), 184-186.

O'Hallaren, B. Nobody (in TV) loves you when you're old and gray. *New York Times,* July 24, 1977, p. 21.

Peterson, M. The visibility and image of old people on television. *Journalism Quarterly,* 1973, *50*(3), 569-573.

Rubin, A.M. Directions in television and aging research. *Journal of Broadcasting,* 1982, *26*(2), 537-551.

Signorielli. N. Marital status in TV drama: A case of reduced options. *Journal of Broadcasting,* 1982, *26*(2), 585-598.

Signorielli, N. *Men and women in television drama: The use of two multivariate techniques for isolating dimensions of characterization.* Doctoral dissertation, University of Pennsylvania, 1975.

Signorielli, N. Patterns in prime time. *Journal of Communication,* 1974. *24*(2), 119-124.

Signorielli, N. *The valuation of occupations on television.* Paper presented at Public Views of Doctors and Lawyers, A National Invitational Conference, The Annenberg School of Communications, University of Pennsylvania, October 18-19, 1979.

Department of Health, Education and Welfare, Public Health Service. *Healthy people: The surgeon general's report on health promotion and disease prevention.* Washington, D.C.: Government Printing Office, 1979.

Older Women and Informal Supports: Impact on Prevention

Jean K. Quam

ABSTRACT. This paper briefly reviews the literature about friendship as an informal support for older women, an at-risk population whose numbers are increasing. Data from an AOA supported study indicate that older women use their friends differentially depending both on the nature and qualities of the friendship as well as the type of help that is required. Friends are more likely to provide help with social-emotional tasks than instrumental ones. Programs should be designed that maximize interaction among older women and those who could serve as informal supports.

Demographic trends alone should prompt practitioners to become better attuned to the particular needs and circumstances of older women. The number of older women in this country has been increasing dramatically. Regardless of the reality of this phenomenon, it has been argued that "the bulk of our attempts at preventive intervention should be focused on the very young" (Shuman & Masterpasqua, 1981, p. 41). For preventive interventionists there is clearly more reason for optimism and long-term benefits in designing programs for children and young adults rather than the elderly. However, older women are clearly an at-risk population in need of the best planning activities and services available.

Currently it is known that older women have a greater probability than older men of being less educated, less financially secure and

Jean K. Quam is an Assistant Professor, School of Social Work, University of Minnesota, Minneapolis.

This research was supported in part by HEW-AOA Grant #90-A-1230 for multidisciplinary research on aging women, awarded to the Faye McBeath Institute on Aging and Adult Life, University of Wisconsin-Madison (1977-1979).

Reprints may be ordered from Jean K. Quam, University of Minnesota, School of Social Work, 400 Ford Hall, Minneapolis, MN 55455.

119

more isolated which contributes to their vulnerability. In addition, over eighty percent of women over age sixty-five have at least one chronic health problem (Block, Davidson, Serock, & Grambs, 1978). Lewis and Butler (1972) state the situation even more pessimistically: "Being an old woman means living alone, on a low or poverty level income, often in substandard housing with inadequate medical care and little chance of employment to supplement resources" (p. 223). Other writers suggest that older women are stigmatized, face the double jeopardy of being both old and female, and enter old age with resignation as a period of non-change and hopelessness (Bell, 1970; Palmore, 1971; Sommers, 1974; Sontag, 1972).

For most older people, "there is great survival value in having someone with whom to share the world—to construct meaning, to provide emotional support" (Hess, 1979, p. 506). Lopata (1975, p. 124) has stated that these supports systems are simply people involved in the "giving and receiving of objects, services, social and emotional supports defined by the receiver and giver as necessary or at least helpful in maintaining a style of life."

Friendships have been defined as an extremely important primary group and potential support system for older women (Adams, 1967; Blau, 1973; Lowenthal, 1975; Quam, 1981). Friendship is defined by Hess (1979, p. 495) as "the quintessential social relationship: voluntary, mutual, enjoyed for its own sake, always in danger of dissolution, dependent upon and illustrative of all levels of social analysis." Because friendship rests on mutual choice and mutual need, it sustains a person's sense of usefulness and self-esteem (Blau, 1973).

Because of increasing numbers of older women living alone and older women who are less likely to remarry after widowhood, it is probable that older women will seek out friendships that could be of critical importance to their satisfaction and happiness in old age. In a review of the literature, Robertson (1978) concluded that "friends act as valuable sources or effective buffers against personal pains produced by major role losses such as widowhood, retirement, divorce or decreased social participation." In defining the functions of friendship, Weis (1969) found intimacy, an opportunity for nurturant behavior, sharing concerns, providing assistance, and reassurance of worth, to be relevant. Intimacy and the capacity for mutuality are important through very old age (Lowenthal, 1975). A person's self image, identity, and attitudes toward herself and others are developed and sustained through friendship (Lowenthal, Thurnher, & Chiriboga, 1977). In addition to intimacy, Robertson and Quam (1979) found assistance and similarity of values and interests to be important dimensions of friendship.

Many studies have tried to compare the supportive functions of family ties to friendship (Adams; 1979; Babchuk, 1965; Cantor, 1979; Paine, 1969). Powers and Bultena (1976) found that older women seemed to distribute their contacts equally among friends, neighbors, children, siblings, spouse, and family, but Wood and Robertson (1978) reported a higher value placed on friendship than on kinship in adult life. Carp (1966) has suggested that friendship may even strengthen family relationships by relieving a burden from kin.

In a study done with elderly in Canada, Peplau (1978) found loneliness associated with less friendship contact, fewer close friends, social anxiety, ineffectiveness in influencing others, low marital satisfaction and life satisfaction, poor health and low income. Townsend (1978) concludes that loneliness is a threat throughout the life cycle but that the risks of aging may increase one's vulnerability to loneliness. Furthermore, Palmore (1980) states that involuntary isolation due to chronic loss of function can be quite stressful, especially among those used to socializing.

As one strategy of preventive intervention, facilitating and strengthening social networks have been shown to reduce morbidity, increase life satisfaction, improve health status and result in more positive mood states (Gottleib, 1981). However, Gottleib (1981) cautions that research simply measuring network size, access and frequency of contact produces data "so general as to be useless" (p. 209). It is critical to analyze the nature and functions of relationships within a network, i.e., friendships, in order to be able to evaluate their usefulness as preventive intervention tools.

This study focuses on the ways in which an older women's friendships serve as a support system. A useful framework is provided by Litwak's theory of shared functions developed in the late 1960s. Litwak proposed that the structure of primary groups and bureaucracies relate to the unique tasks each could best accomplish (Litwak, 1970; Litwak & Figueira, 1968). For example, a primary group because of its small size, face-to-face contact, affectivity and long-term commitments could best handle unanticipated events whereas a bureaucracy is more suited to tasks requiring technically trained experts or large numbers of people. Specifying the functions of a primary group such as friendship more precisely, Dean and Lin (1977) state that there are two major functions that exist. One is an instrumental function which is "geared to the fulfillment of tasks" and the other is an expressive function which is "geared to the satisfaction of needs and the maintenance of solidarity" (p. 407).

To assess what characteristics of a friendship may enhance its preventive function is a difficult task. In the 1950's, British anthropologists (Barnes, 1954; Bott, 1955; Nadel, 1957) introduced the idea of social networks and described the ways in which they promoted supportive activities among the members of the network. Mitchell (1969) felt that the metaphor of social network was analytically useful and expanded on the works of others to identify characteristics of social networks that could also be used to portray the nature and functions of friendships. These included such qualities as intensity, reachability, density, durability, directedness and similarity. Thoits (1982) concluded that to measure and to examine the structural properties of a social support system using classic network indicators as well as the functional properties of the system "directs the researcher's attention to various types, sources and degrees of support received from significant others and to the structural properties of support systems, foci which have been lacking in most previous work" (p. 149).

In order to more fully understand the potential of friendship as a prevention strategy, the functions of the relationship should be explored. Specifically, in this analysis, it is hypothesized that whether or not an older woman chooses a friend to help her or to offer support to her will depend on three categories of independent variables: (1) the structural properties or qualities of the friendship, (2) the specific helping task, and (3) the characteristics of the subject herself (i.e., age, work status, and marital status).

METHODOLOGY

Sample

Subjects were 500 women over age fifty selected using a stratified random sampling procedure. A personal interview was completed by a trained interviewer in the subject's home. In addition, a self-administered questionnaire was left with the subject and picked up later by the interviewer. The initial instrument contained demographic questions regarding singlehood, family relationships, friendship, physical activity, work history, health, and organizational political activity. One year later, in the summer of 1979, the same women were contacted again to be interviewed in their homes a second time. At this point there were four hundred women remaining in the study due to subjects moving away, dying, and refusing to participate a second time. The focus of the second interview was the self and social connectedness. This interview sought information specifically looking for changes from the previous year and measured the subject's participation in social service programs, health, feelings about death and dying, friendships, social connections, and marriage life satisfaction. The findings in this study are based on the interviews conducted in the second year.

Table 1 presents the most salient demographic characteristics of this sample of older women. The average respondent in this study was a white women in her late sixties ($m = 66$ years) who was in good health and felt she was satisfied with her life. Slightly over half of the women were living with their spouses or other family members, and most continued to remain in their own homes (65%). As expected with this age group, approximately one-third were widowed and another eleven percent had never married. Although subjects defined themselves as "middle-class," the average household was slightly over $16,000 a year. With the exception of a somewhat higher income and more education, this sample was fairly representative of older women in general.

The subject's support system consisted of a very large extended family system, i.e., grandchildren, aunts, cousins, nephews ($M = 17.4$ family members, range $= 1$–132), with a relatively large number of casual friends and acquaintances ($M = 44$ friends, range $= 0$–1000), and a somewhat smaller circle of close friends ($M = 4$ close friends, range $= 0$–30). The average number of close friends was less than that found in other friendship studies in which the average was about six friends for women throughout the lifecycle (Lowenthal, Thurnher, & Chiriboga, 1977). Most of the women had at least a few friends living within their own neighborhood (76%) and most of the women felt they had enough friends (78%). Despite the fact that these subjects appeared to have extensive support networks, when asked what they considered to be "the most important problem older women are faced with in our society," they overwhelmingly responded with concerns of "loneliness," "loss of friends/spouse," and "not being needed" (40%).

Table 1

Demographic Characteristics of Study Group

Variable	Number	Percent
Age (by decade)	n	%
50's	107	26.8
60's	164	41.1
70's	93	23.3
80's	32	8.0
90's	3	.8
Total	399	100.0
Life Satisfaction		
Very Dissatisfied	10	2.6
Somewhat Dissatisfied	41	10.6
Somewhat Satisfied	152	39.3
Very Satisfied	154	39.8
Completely Satisfied	30	7.7
Total	387	100.0
Health		
Very poor	4	1.0
Poor	11	2.7
Fair	88	22.2
Good	193	48.4
Excellent	103	25.7
Total	399	100.0
Marital Status		
Married	190	47.5
Widowed	128	32.0
Single	44	11.0
Divorced	35	8.8
Separated	3	.7
Total	400	100.0
Living Situation		
Live alone	172	43.1
Live with spouse	190	47.6
Live with others	37	9.3
Total	399	100.0

Measures

The independent variables included those qualities that have been used to explicate one's social network by Mitchell (1969) and others. These characteristics were used to explore the possibility that they could measure the rather abstract concept of friendship. Specifically, the qualities and some of the indicators that were used include: (1) intensity or the strength and importance of the friendship (i.e., "If something were to happen to change or disrupt the friendship how distressing would this be?"), (2) reachability or the access one has to a friend (i.e., proximity, frequency of contact in person and by telephone), (3) density (i.e., "Does your friend know your other friends?"), (4) directedness or the degree of equity in the friendship ("When you think about how much you do for your friend. . .how do things stack up?"), (5) durability or the meaningfulness of friendship over time (i.e., "Do you think your friendship is more meaningful now than it was ten years ago?"), and (6) similarity, defined both objectively (age and sex) and subjectively (attitudes, values, interests and mutual activities). In an earlier analysis of these women (Robertson & Quam, 1979) which looked at the nature of friendship, it was found that other than age and marital status, demographic variables seemed to make very little difference in the way in which an older women selected their friends. Thus, the only variables that were included in this analysis were age, marital status and work status (which approached significance in the previous study).

Litwak (1970) found that there are many "non-expert" tasks that untrained people such as friends can handle. In previous studies, hypothetical situations have been designed such that subjects can consider who they would turn to for help without actually being involved in a real situation (Cantor, 1979; Rosow, 1967). In the present study, a series of twenty vignettes describing experiences that could realistically occur in the life of an older women were used. Subjects were instructed as follows:

> Now, I'm going to describe a situation that might arise and ask you who, if anyone, you would turn to. Even though you think a particular situation is unlikely to occur to you, try to think about what you'd do if it did happen. Who would you first turn to? Your family? Friends? Other resources in the community?

The vignettes were grouped into two general types of tasks: (1) instrumental tasks including financial assistance and advice and general assistance (i.e., transportation, help when ill), and (2) expressive tasks including confiding in a friend about personal problems (i.e., daughter's divorce, husband's illness) and enjoyment (i.e., going on a trip, taking a walk, discussing a book). The dependent variables were the responses to these vignettes which were classified into two groups: (1) those subjects stating that they would first turn to a friend for help in these situations, and (2) those subjects who would turn to people other than friends for help (i.e., family, professionals).

To determine differences between those older women who use their friends as support systems and those who do not, a multivariate model of discriminant analysis was utilized. Discriminant analysis is a regression equation with a dependent variable that represents membership as expressed by a nominal variable (in this instance the variable is the use or non-use of friends). As a technique it differentiates the two groups by finding a linear combination of variables that best discriminates the users of friends from the non-users. The coefficients indicate the relative importance of each variable in the discrimination process and can be interpreted similarly to beta's in multiple regression. A discriminant analysis was completed on each of the five sub-categories comprising both the instrumental and expressive functions of friendship.

RESULTS

Choosing a friend for support varied according to the type of help that was needed. Friends were least likely to be viewed as a resource for the more instrumental tasks of financial and general assistance (15.7% and 26.3% respectively). However, on the expressive tasks, older women relied on friends to listen to both their personal (39.7%) and their family problems (31.2%). Subjects were most likely to select a friend (64.2%) as opposed to selecting anyone else 35.8%) for enjoyment (Table 2).

Results indicated that network variables describing the nature of friendship as well as demographic variables about the subject were able to distinguish between older women who chose friends for support and those who chose someone else. The most important factor in characterizing who would select a friend for financial help or ad-

Table 2

Percentage of Subjects Choosing a Friend or Other
Support Person According to Type of Helping Task

I. Instrumental Tasks

   A. Task: General Assistance

Support Person	n	%
Friend	105	26.3
Other	295	73.7

   B. Task: Financial Assistance and Advice

   Support Person

Friend	63	15.7
Other	337	84.3

II. Expressive Tasks

   A. Task: Confide Regarding Personal Problems

   Support Person

Friend	159	39.7
Other	241	60.3

   B. Task: Confide Regarding Family Problems

   Support Person

Friend	125	31.2
Other	275	68.8

   C. Task: Enjoyment

   Support Person

Friend	257	64.2
Other	143	35.8

   Total N = 400

vice was age. Those who were younger, i.e., less than age sixty-five, were more likely to turn to friends. Having a friend who was readily available and in close contact was also an important variable. Somewhat less important was having an intense friendship and not being married. Eighty-four percent of the cases were correctly classified by the discriminant function. Not being married, having an intense friendship and being younger were also associated with choosing a friend for the tasks labeled "general assistance." Adding two other qualities of the friendship—high durability and high reachability—led to seventy-five percent of the cases being correctly classified (Table 3).

For the expressive categories, differences emerged according to the nature of the task. A subject who was younger, not married, but still working was most likely to confide in her friends regarding both family and personal problems. Also, the friendship was perceived of as an intense one. In discussing personal problems, the support person was more likely to be in regular contact with the subject and to be part of a dense friendship network. However, similarity of attitudes, values and interests was a more important factor when discussing family problems. The combinations of these factors presented in Table 4 produced 69% of the subjects correctly classified according to sharing family problems and 65% correctly classified for tasks related to sharing personal problems.

Choice of a friend for enjoyment, another expressive function, was strongly related to marital status. Qualities of the friendship such as seeing one's friend regularly, durability, intensity and subjective similarity (age and sex), when added to the marital status variable, produced a correct classification of sixty-nine percent of the subjects.

DISCUSSION

For older women, an at-risk population within our society whose numbers are increasing, friends clearly serve as a source of support. The findings suggest that friends are more likely to perform expressive functions rather than instrumental ones. Asking for financial advice, borrowing money or needing transportation may be needs that can be met more effectively by formalized social services or family members. However, as suggested in much of the literature, peers are important sources of age-role and sex-role modeling, informal counseling and advice giving. In this study, older women actively sought out friends for socialization and for their expressive needs.

Primary prevention as a relatively new area of practice suggests that intervention can strengthen an at-risk population's immunity and resistance to problems. Can friends perform such a function? Can they prevent loneliness and dependency and enhance one's ability to resist the assaults of the aging process? Our knowledge of

Table 3

Variables Related to Choosing a Friend as a Support
Person for Instrumental Tasks

Instrumental Tasks

A. Financial Assistance and Advice

Related Variables	Standardized DF Coefficient (N = 353)
Less Than Age 65	.65 *
High Reachability	.41
More Intense Friendship	.35
Not Married	.35
Canonical Correlation	.19
% Correctly Classified	84.2%

B. General Assistance

Related Variables	Standardized DF Coefficient (N = 353)
Not Married	.63 **
More Intense Friendship	.51 ***
Less Than Age 65	.41
More Durable Friendship	.35 ***
High Reachability	.32
Canonical Correlation	.35
% Correctly Classified	75.2%

NOTE: Since the direction of the meaning of each variables' effect is stated in words, signs are omitted from the coefficients to avoid confusion.

*p <.05

**p <.01

***p <.001

129

Table 4

Variables Related to Choosing a Friend as a Support Person for Expressive Tasks

Expressive Tasks

A. Confiding Regarding Family Problems

Related Variables	Standardized DF Coefficient (N=353)	
Less Than Age 65	.53	**
Similar Attitudes, Values & Interests	.42	**
Not Married	.35	
More Intense Friendship	.30	*
Working	.29	**
Canonical Correlation	.33	
% Correctly Classified	69.2%	

B. Confiding Regarding Personal Problems

Related Variables	Standardized DF Coefficient (N=353)	
Less Than Age 65	.52	*
More Intense Friendship	.48	**
Hear from Friend Frequently	.43	*
Not Married	.40	
Working	.29	*
High Density of Friends	.27	*
Canonical Correlation	.28	
% Correctly Classified	65.5%	

C. Enjoyment

Related Variables	Standardized DF Coefficient (N=353)	
Not Married	.88	***
See More Frequently	.33	
More Durable Friendship	.32	***
More Intense Friendship	.27	**
Similar Age & Sex of Friend	.19	
Canonical Correlation	.40	
% Correctly Classified	69.7%	

Note: Since the direction of the meaning of each variables' effect is stated in words, signs are omitted from the coefficients to avoid confusion.

*p < .05

** p < .01

*** p < .001

the older woman has led to the identification of times in her development that are particularly stressful and place her in a vulnerable position. Block et al. (1978) identified six of these situations: postparental years, widowhood, divorce, retirement, change in health status, and institutionalization. To this list could be added the loss of a friend and a move to a new living situation. These are times in which the support of friends is valuable if friendship networks are well developed and functioning smoothly. In fact, friends may also perform secondary and tertiary prevention functions by helping to identify problems and needs for services as they occur and encouraging treatment as well as helping to keep a problem from becoming worse after it has occurred.

As a strategy for prevention, encouraging the supportive qualities of informal helpers, particularly friends, should be considered. Friendship is an invaluable resource to maintain independence, promote self-esteem, provide role-modeling and encouraging activities for older women. Gilbert (1982) cautions that with all the attention that primary prevention has drawn, practitioners need to carefully and critically explore the uncertainty that exists between its implicit promises and its applicability, especially in an area as unexplored as friendship.

Practitioners, planners and policy-makers need to determine what can be handled informally and what may be more appropriate for formalized prevention services. They need to realize what this study has suggested—that in addition to instrumental needs, older women have needs for socialization and intimacy. Snow and Gordon (1980) point out the inadequacies of social policies affecting the elderly which have overlooked this fact. These policies are reflected in "transportation policies in which one can get a minibus for health but not for social purposes; or in the nature and location of housing which leads to social isolation; or in limited alternatives to institutionalization making it difficult or impossible to support the individual in situations closer to family and social ties" (p. 466). Prevention programs can be designed that maximize interaction among older women and their friends, family and neighbors.

REFERENCES

Adams, B. N. Interaction theory and social network. *Sociometry,* 1967, *30,* 64-78.
Adams, B. N. Isolation, function and beyond: American kinship in the 1960's. *Journal of Marriage and the Family,* 1970, *32* 575-597.
Babchuk, N. Primary friends and kin: A study of the associations of middle class couples. *Social Forces,* 1965, *43,* 483-493.

Barnes, J. A. Class and committees in a Norweigan island parish. *Human Relations,* 1954, *7,* 39-58.

Bell, I. P. The double standard. *Transaction,* 1970, *8,* 75-80.

Blau, Z. *Old age in a changing society.* New York: Franklin Watts, 1973.

Block, M. R., Davidson, J. L., Serock. K. E., & Grambs, J. D. *Uncharted territory: Issues and concerns of women over 40.* College Park, Maryland: University of Maryland, 1978.

Bott, E. *Family and social network.* London: Tavistock Publications, 1951.

Cantor, M. H. Neighbors and friends: An overlooked resource in the informal support system. *Research on Aging,* 1979, *1,* 434-463.

Carp, F. M. *Patterns of living and housing of middle-aged and older adults.* Washington, D.C.: Government Printing Office, 1966.

Dean, A., & Lin, N. The stress-buffering role of social support: Problems and prospects for systematic investigation. *Journal of Nervous and Mental Disease,* 1977, *165,* 403-417.

Gilbert, N. Policy issues in primary prevention. *Social Work,* 1982, *27,* 293-297.

Gottleib, B. Preventive interventions involving social networks and social supports. In B. Gottleib (Ed.), *Social networks and social support.* Beverly Hills: Sage, 1981.

Hess, B. B. Sex roles, friendship and the life course. *Research on Aging,* 1979, *1,* 494-515.

Lewis, M. I., & Butler, R. N. Why is women's lib ignoring old women? *Aging and Human Development,* 1972, *3,* 223-231.

Litwak, E. *The scholarly practitioner: A collection of papers.* Report No. ESEA, Title 5. Champaign, Illinois: University of Illinois, 1970.

Litwak, E., & Figueira, J. Technological innovation and theoretical functions of primary groups and bureaucratic structures. *American Journal of Sociology,* 1968, *73,* 468-481.

Lopata, H. Z. Widowhood: Societal factors in life-span disruptions and alternatives. In N. Datan & L. H. Ginsberg (Eds.), *Life-span developmental psychology.* New York: Academic Press, 1975.

Lowenthal, M. F. Psychosocial variations across the adult life course. *Gerontologist,* 1975, *15,* 6-12.

Lowenthal, M. F., Thurnher, M., & Chiriboga, D. *Four stages of life.* Washington, D.C.: Jossey-Bass, 1977.

Mitchell, J. C. *Social networks in urban areas.* Manchester, England: Manchester University Press, 1969.

Nadel, S. F. *The theory of social structure.* London: Cohen & West, 1957.

Paine, R. In search of friendship: An exploratory analysis in middle class culture. *Man,* 1969, *4,* 505-524.

Palmore, E. Variables related to needs of the aged poor. *Journal of Gerontology,* 1971, *26,* 524-531.

Palmore, E. The social factors in aging. In E. W. Busse & D. G. Glazer (Eds.), *Handbook of geriatric psychiatry.* New York: Van Nostrand Reinhold, 1980.

Peplau, L. Loneliness: A cognitive analysis. *Essence,* 1978, *2,* 207-220.

Powers, E. A., & Bultena, G. L. Sex differences in intimate friendships in old age. *Journal of Marriage and the Family,* 1976, *38,* 739-747.

Quam, J. K. *The utility of friendship for older women: An application of the task-specific model.* Unpublished doctoral dissertation, University of Wisconsin-Madison, 1981.

Robertson, J. F. Women in mid-life: Crises, reverberations and support networks. *The Family Coordinator,* 1978, *6,* 375-382.

Robertson, J. F., & Quam, J. K. *The essence of friendship in adult life.* Paper presented at the Western Gerontological Meeting, San Francisco, California, 1979.

Rosow, I. *Social integration of the aged.* New York: The Free Press, 1967.

Shurman, B. J., & Masterpasqua, F. Preventive intervention during the perinatal and infancy periods: Overview and guidelines for evaluation. *Prevention in Human Services,* 1981, *1,* 41-57.

Snow, D. L., & Gordon, J. B. Social network analysis and intervention with the elderly. *The Gerontologist,* 1980, *20,* 463-467.

Sommers, T. The compounding impact of age on sex: Another dimension of the double standard. *Civil Rights Digest*, 1974, 7, 3-9.

Sontag, S. The double standard of aging. *Saturday Review*, 1972, 55, 29-38.

Thoits, P. A. Conceptual, methodological and theoretical problems in studying social support as a buffer against life stress. *Journal of Health and Social Behavior*, 1982, 23, 145-159.

Townsend, P. Isolation and loneliness in the aged. *Essence*, 1978, 2, 221-237.

Weiss, R. S. The fund of sociability. *Transaction*, 1969, 6, 36-43.

Wood, V., & Robertson, J. F. Friendship and kinship interaction: Differential effects on the morale of the elderly. *Journal of Marriage and the Family*, 1978, 40, 367-375.

Opportunities for Prevention
of Domestic Neglect and Abuse
of the Elderly

Richard L. Douglass

ABSTRACT. Recent research has demonstrated that domestic neglect and abuse of the elderly is not uncommon in the United States. It is a social problem that has not been extensively researched, however. One of the few studies, conducted in Michigan, found that the oldest and most frail elderly were a target group of elevated risk. Victims of neglect or abuse tend to be living with adult children or other informal caretakers who become neglectful or abusive when the burdens of providing care for a frail, elderly person interact with stress, little or no preparation for providing personal care over a long time span, medical problems of the caretaker, alcohol abuse, financial difficulties, and other situational factors. Family histories of neglect or abuse and other causal hypotheses have also been investigated. Recent studies are reviewed and found to be in general agreement regarding the nature and apparent dynamics of this emerging problem among the elderly. Opportunities for prevention are discussed in terms of current models of service to the aging and redirection of other public health and social services.

No references to research on domestic neglect or abuse of the elderly could be found in the gerontological literature prior to 1975 when Burston, an English emergency room physician, suggested that the elderly were occasionally subjected to mistreatment by family members providing their care. Burston's letter in the *British Medical Journal* (Burston, 1975) was largely unnoticed until it was discovered by social scientists in the United States between 1978 and 1980. As reported by Cronin and Allen (1982), research on neglect and abuse of the elderly between 1978 and 1980 identified and provided preliminary measurement of a hitherto unacknowledged social

Requests for reprints may be sent to Richard L. Douglass, Institute on Aging, Jewish Home for Aged, 19100 West Seven Mile Road, Detroit, MI 48219.

135

problem. The initial studies of the problem enjoyed a rapid acceptance by service providers, legislators, and academic researchers; however, the existing literature is still very small and exploratory in nature.

This paper will review the state of knowledge of domestic neglect and abuse of the elderly and relate this new information to the opportunities that exist for prevention. Rather than proposing a new system of agencies, policies, laws, and specialists in the field, it will be suggested that human services can take advantage of existing services and models of service delivery to prevent the prevalence and incidence of domestic mistreatment of the elderly from approaching the scale of such problems with children and spouses.

In 1978 Steinmetz presented case histories of abuse and other mistreatment of the elderly before the U.S. House of Representatives Select Committee on Aging (Select Committee on Aging, 1980a). Concurrent with Steinmetz's work in Delaware, Rathbone-McCuan was investigating cases of abuse which emerged from hospital emergency rooms in St. Louis, Missouri (Rathbone-McCuan, 1980). Both of these efforts produced descriptive studies of elderly persons who were abused, exploited or neglected by the people they depended upon. The critical role of such pilot efforts cannot be overstated. While such research and case analysis may not be sufficient to formulate program design or social policy, it is such work that stimulates more systematic and generalizable research. Early case exploration raises the consciousness of laymen and professionals and suggests hypotheses for subsequent research to pursue.

Lau and Kosberg, in Cleveland, Ohio, reviewed records of 400 consecutive admissions of elderly patients at the Cleveland Chronic Disease Center (Lau & Kosberg, 1978). The purpose of their review was to determine if any evidence of neglect or abuse of patients could be found in the records or in the recollections of assigned case workers. Lau and Kosberg concluded that "a significant proportion" of these elderly had been neglected or physically abused prior to their admission to the Chronic Disease Center. The conclusion was extended to suggest that the sources of such mistreatment were the informal caretakers of the elderly patients.

During the 1978-1979 time period two studies were conducted which utilized mail questionnaires to samples of professionals regarding their knowledge of abuse or neglect of the elderly. O'Malley and her colleagues mailed questionnaires to a variety of direct service personnel throughout Massachusetts with an emphasis on private agency staff, nurses, police, hospital social workers, and legal aid workers (O'Malley, Segars, Perez, Mitchell, & Kneupfel, 1979.) This study's principal finding was that a wide variety of professionals did experience cases of neglect or abuse of dependent elderly. Victims were generally found to be older than non-victimized elderly and were also more frail, mentally or physically disabled, female, and living with the person responsible for the mistreatment. The authors noted that the caretakers were usually expressing some form of acute stress such as drinking problems or drug abuse, serious medical conditions, or financial difficulties. There was a positive association with the level of responsibility for the aged dependent and the likelihood of neglect or abuse. This latter conclusion has been repeatedly noted in this young literature. Rathbone-McCuan and Hashimi (1982, Chapter 8), for instance, focused on the isolation of the caretakers and victims alike as a source of stress and a key element in the social etiology of neglect or abuse. In the Congressional Hearings sponsored by the Select Committee on Aging, the stress of caring for a highly dependent, elderly person was noted to be accelerated when coupled with external stress, financial insufficiency, marital problems, or other domestic issues (Select Committee on Aging, 1980b).

The most significant methodological problem with the study of O'Malley and her colleagues was its undersampling of caseworkers and protective service specialists in public agencies. Their emphasis on the private sector probably imposed a bias in the direction of smaller routine caseloads among the sample's respondents and, possibly, a generally higher socio-economic status of the respondents' clients and patients.

The other mail survey was conducted as part of a larger project by Block and Sinnott at the University of Maryland (Block & Sinnott, 1979). These investigators mailed questionnaires to members of the Gerontological Society of America, the American Psychological Association, and the College of Emergency Physicians who resided in Maryland. Block and Sinnott found that 13.4% of their respondents reported familiarity with at least one case of neglect, abuse, or financial exploitation of an aged dependent by that person's caretakers. A range of physical abuse, neglect, and exploitation was described which concurred with the results of the work of other contributors. Block and Sinnott reported that the most prevalent form of mistreatment was what they called "psychological abuse."

The Maryland study, despite its concurrence with other studies, had a low response rate (under 33%) and it is uncertain that the membership of professional organizations as broadly represented as the American Psychological Association is an appropriate sampling frame for an exploration of this particular problem area. The authors' conclusions regarding the relative prevalence of neglect, however, were important and were substantiated by the field study conducted in Michigan.

Douglass, Hickey, and Noel (1980) directed an exploratory study in 1978-1979 in response to their hypothesis that because the frail, dependent elderly present many of the same vulnerabilities that are associated with dependent children, it is reasonable to expect some forms of mistreatment in certain situations and circumstances. The Michigan study was conducted at the same time as the work noted above and was, therefore, similarly unaffected by the approaches or findings of any previous research regarding domestic mistreatment of the elderly.

STUDY SITES AND PARTICIPANTS

Personal interviews were conducted with community professionals in five locations in Michigan, including two rural counties, two small city/suburban counties, and the city of Detroit. Initial samples were taken from lists of community professionals in each study location and included individuals who were predominantly involved with serving the elderly. Interviews with these initial respondents provided nominations of other community professionals which led to a peer nomination sample in each study site. While this method of respondent selection has many of the obvious limitations of a quota sample, and no small threat of self-selection, it was considered to be an efficient approach for an exploratory field study. Principal respondent screening requirements were that at least one-third of the respondents' routine activities must be spent in direct service delivery with the elderly, and administrative or supervisory personnel were to be excluded whenever possible. Some categories of respondents, such as police, clergy, and morticians, could not be held to this criteria as they served large, multigeneration populations. The respondents were about equally divided between the public and the private service sectors which differs from the O'Malley et al. study. Respondents in the Michigan study included police officers and detectives, physicians in general and family practice, nurses and aids in public and home health care, social workers in medical or outreach services, adult protective service workers, community mental health workers, lawyers, aging services workers, clergy, morticians, coroners, and medical examiners. Aging services workers included the staff of congregate meal sites and senior citizens centers, and outreach workers in Area Agencies on Aging. The distribution of respondents by category is shown in Table 1.

Two hundred and seventy interviews were conducted of which 228 were included in statistical analyses. The remaining 42 interviews were with individuals whose work did not fit into any obvious category or whose work was predominantly devoted to advocacy at the public policy level. Some of the interviews not included in the statistical analysis were with respondents with unique perspectives such as Probate Judges; however, the small number of such respondents suggested that even the most simple descriptive statistics would be misleading when combined with similar calculations from other larger respondent groups. Information from these outlying interviews were helpful in contextual interpretation and in anecdotal examples of cases of mistreatment or potential changes in public policy.

Table 1

Distribution of Respondents by
Professional/Occupational Category

Respondent Category	N	%
Police officers and detectives	25	11.9
Physicians in general and family practice	18	7.9
Nurses and aides in public and home health	27	11.8
Social workers in medical, outreach services	40	17.5
Adult protective service workers	21	9.2
Community mental health workers	16	7.0
Attorneys	17	7.5
Aging services workers	17	7.5
Clergy	24	10.5
Morticians, coroners, medical examiners	23	10.0
TOTAL	228	(100.0)

PROCEDURE

Data were collected in personal interviews at the work settings of respondents. Interviews were structured to provide flexibility according to the actual experiences of respondents with neglect or abuse of the elderly. Interviews with respondents who had little or no knowledge of specific cases were relatively brief with basic information collected about the respondent, his/her agency's capability of handling cases of mistreatment, and attitudes regarding the general status of informal home care of dependent elderly. When respondents indicated that they were knowledgeable regarding neglect or abuse of the elderly, contingency questions permitted the interviewer to pursue these areas in considerable detail. All interviews were tape-recorded and fully transcribed to provide an exact record of responses to open-ended questions, relevant stray remarks and elaborations of certain questions which were structured to elicit considerable details of specific cases of mistreatment, casefinding methods, or community resources which were useful to respondents when dealing with neglect or abuse of the elderly.

The Michigan study placed major emphasis on three basic questions: Is there neglect or abuse of the elderly in the community? What are the characteristics of such mistreatment, if it exists? What community professionals or agencies respond to cases of mistreatment and what do they do when cases are reported?

The questionnaire was designed to guide the interview through several specific categories of information, including:

1. Information about the respondents and their professional involvement with the elderly;
2. Perceived degree to which daily needs are met by informal caretakers upon whom the elderly depend;
3. Perceptions regarding relative frequency and characteristics of different manifestations of neglect or abuse;
4. Case finding procedures;
5. Reporting and intervention procedures.

In an attempt to organize respondents' independent perceptions of neglect or abuse, four categories of mistreatment were defined and measured separately. Only respondents with direct experience with some form of mistreatment were asked questions about these manifestations of neglect or abuse. The four categories were:

1. *Passive Neglect*—when a dependent elder is left unattended, ignored, or isolated, or unintentionally not provided with essential goods or services;
2. *Active Neglect*—when a dependent elder is intentionally unattended, ignored, or isolated, or when essential goods or services such as assistance to the bathroom, medicine, food, or exercise are withheld;
3. *Verbal or Emotional Abuse*—when a dependent elder is called names, insulted, treated like a child, frightened, humiliated, intimidated, or threatened;
4. *Physical Abuse*—when a dependent elder is hit, slapped, bruised, burned, sexually molested or attacked, cut, or physically restrained.

RESULTS

Of the 228 respondents used for the principal analyses, 156 (68%) were knowledgeable about specific cases of neglect or abuse in the 12 months preceding the interview. These respondents provided information on questions regarding acknowledged direct case experience. One hundred twenty-five (54%) of the respondents expressed the opinion that while the basic needs of the elderly were usually met, the people responsible for the elderly in their care were often poorly prepared for such a task due to inadequate knowledge or understanding of the specific problems of the aged. Sixty respondents (23%) related that the needs of the elderly were sometimes unmet because the people responsible for daily care felt frustrated, overwhelmed, overly stressed, or burdened. A smaller number of respondents, 41 (18%), reported that when needs were unmet, sometimes it was because the caretaker was too busy or too uncaring to fulfill the role. In addition, when the general condition of the elderly was discussed, a tendency of respondents was to conclude that when needs were *not* met, the aged were often also treated like children or in other ways which reduced their feelings of self worth.

The question which dealt with case experiences with passive neglect was stated as: "To what extent are vulnerable adults (aged) unintentionally ignored, left alone, physically isolated, or forgotten by those upon whom they depend?" More respondents, 150 (66%), reported knowledge of this form of mistreatment than any other form. Ninety-seven percent of these respondents indicated that isolation was a problem of great concern to them and that they knew of instances of unintentional isolation which resulted in harm to elderly dependents. Many of these respondents also specified that families were simply too busy or too concerned with their own lives to adequately pay attention to dependent elderly. Forty percent of these 150 respondents indicated that families who had responsibilities for an aged relative were often unskilled, lacked education, or lacked knowledge, understanding, or awareness of the specific needs of frail elderly people. One hundred three respondents regarded passive neglect as a consequence of aged dependents being the responsibility of family members who, themselves, were elderly, frail, or chronically ill. Few respondents (6) who knew of cases of other forms of neglect or abuse were not also aware of cases of passive neglect.

The question on active neglect was stated as: "To what extent are vulnerable adults (aged) *intentionally* kept from receiving the things they need?" Of the 93 respondents (41%) who identified active neglect, 64% of the areas of neglect included forced confinement, isolation, withholding of food, or withholding of medications. The majority of the respondents' comments reiterated statements made earlier; however, forced confinement was only mentioned by these respondents.

One hundred four respondents (46%) responded affirmatively to the question, "To what extent are vulnerable adults (aged) verbally or emotionally abused by those upon whom they depend?" Forty-six of these respondents indicated that dependent elderly were frequently treated in a manner which diminished their personal identity and dignity as well as their feelings of self worth. One hundred and twelve respondents indicated that dependent elderly are often threatened, "talked down to," treated like children or in a condescending manner, or called names. Also, the nurses and caseworkers in the sample were particularly aware of verbal and emotional abuse in terms of overprotection and denial of the need of frail elderly to be independent to the fullest extent possible. Further discussion indicated that verbally or emotionally abused elderly are frequently over-supervised and removed as active participants from decision-making concerning their own lives, including decisions about their financial affairs.

The question which dealt with physical abuse was stated as: "To what extent are vulnerable adults (aged) physically abused?" Most respondents did not recall experiences with serious physical abuse. However, 64 respondents (28%) had some experiences with physical abuse cases. In addition, 80 respondents (35%) suspected physical abuse in the context of cases of neglect or verbal/emotional abuse while having no direct evidence to support their suspicions. Those respondents who had actual experience with physical abuse tended to mention possible causes in their discussions related to this question. The emotional or personal problems of the caretaker in dealing with the needs of a dependent older person, the problem of stubbornness and unwillingness to accept dependency on the part of the victim, or alcohol abuse of one or both parties surfaced most frequently. Respondents were generally able to provide explicit details of forms of violence and the consequences of such acts on the frail elderly and were concerned that emergency medical services were infrequently sensitive to the causes of traumatic injuries among older people which result from physical abuse.

Three sets of questions were designed to elicit information concerning the causes of neglect and abuse. The first means of identifying causal factors was simply to ask each respondent what he or she considered the causes of neglect and abuse to be. The second question was, "In the situations with which you are familiar, are the causes of neglect different from the causes of abuse?" The forced response portions of each answer included valid *yes, no, a matter of degree,* and *don't know* categories. Respondents were asked to elaborate on their answers.

The final question regarding the causes of neglect and abuse of the elderly required each respondent to consider four alternative causal hypotheses:

1. A person who relies on someone else for his or her care is more likely to be neglected and/or abused;
2. A child who is abused or witnesses abuse grows up to be an abusive adult;
3. Life crises in either the abused or the abuser trigger abusive behavior;
4. Environmental factors such as a crowded living space or physical isolation play a major part in bringing about neglectful or abusive behavior.

After considering each of these possible hypotheses, each respondent was asked to select, in their opinion, the "most important."

The basis of this decision was the respondent's individual interpretation. When elaborating on their answer to the question of the causes of neglect or abuse being similar or different, the most frequently cited remark dealt with the distinction between intentional and unintentional behaviors toward an older person which resulted in neglect or abuse. Some respondents used the term "motive or the absence of motive" when distinguishing between neglect or abuse. These respondents were also likely to disagree with the active and passive neglect categories used in the study questionnaire. Most respondents, however, generally considered abuse to be the result of an intentional set of behaviors. Neglect, on the other hand, was considered to be intentional by as many respondents as thought it to be unintentional. This supports the conceptual distinction between passive and active neglect.

The distributions among professional categories of responses to the question which asked them to select the "most important" of four alternative causal hypotheses in part was interpreted to reflect the variation in training and professional experience of the different groups of respondents. A clear pattern of selection regarding the hypotheses may reflect the fact that most professionals do not see clients or patients in a truly holistic way, but tend to address their emotional, physical, or legal problems separately.

Hypothesis 1, which dealt with levels of dependency, was the clear choice of lawyers, employees of congregate meal sites and senior citizens' centers, and aging services outreach workers. Hypothesis 2, which suggested that abused children could become abusive adult caretakers, was selected as the most important by police, nurses, physicians, and morticians. Life crises were considered a cause of mistreatment in the third hypothesis. Life crises were seen as the most important of the alternative causal hypotheses by mental health workers. Lastly, the fourth hypothesis, which concerned environmental factors, was selected by social services caseworkers.

Principal causal factors which were suggested by respondents included lack of sufficient financial resources, alcohol or drug abuse, lack of community service resources as alternatives to family care, emotional disturbances of the caretaker, long-term hostility between the aged dependent and the caretaker, high levels of physical and emotional dependency of the aged person, and a prospect of increasing dependency over an extended period of time. Thrity-eight percent of the respondents reported that abused people feared reprisals from the perpetrator/caretaker if the mistreatment was reported to authorities. This was viewed as a form of abuse in itself in that the feared consequences of reporting were increased abuse, withholding of food, clothing, shelter, or companionship, or abandonment. It was noted by 28% of the respondents, in various statements, that mistreatment of an aged person could be the continuation of long-standing abusiveness among family members and may not necessarily suggest increased vulnerability of an aging person within the family.

The victims, themselves, were considered to be at least partially responsible for their own mistreatment by 21% of the respondents. The victims' "difficult" personalities, levels of dependency, or personal habits were considered to be frequent causes of neglect or abuse. One specific contributing cause of physical abuse was alcohol abuse of the victim, the perpetrator, or both, which was indicated by half of all respondents who had professional experience with physical abuse of an aged person.

Each respondent who reported some experience with neglect or abuse was asked about the average incidence of such mistreatment that came to their attention in a typical month. In general, passive neglect and verbal or emotional abuse were far more frequently encountered by respondents than the other kinds of mistreatment. Respondents affiliated with services to the aging and caseworkers were most likely to encounter passive neglect and verbal or emotional abuse with over 20 cases in a typical month. Active neglect was most frequently encountered by lawyers, aging services workers, and caseworkers. Physical abuse was most often experienced in a typical month by police officers, caseworkers, and mental health counselors. The incidence of all categories of mistreatment was low when compared to the samples total client, patient, or public contact in a month. At least one respondent in each category encountered some neglect or abuse, with the exception of physical abuse, in an average month.

DISCUSSION

The research between 1978 and 1980 verified that all is not well in the homes of many elderly who are highly dependent upon adult children, grandchildren, or other informal caretakers. Relative prevalence, according to most authors suggests that neglect and emotional types of abuse are considerably more widespread than physical abuse. In the Michigan study, passive neglect was the most frequently cited by community professionals. No research has yet measured the true incidence or prevalence, however, and all studies thus far have had considerable limitations of design, instrumentation, response rates, and conceptualization. All of the studies to date have been considered to be exploratory by both the investigators and their sponsors.

Given that the state of knowledge is limited, it is, nevertheless, possible to recognize some common denominators which can be viewed as hopeful signs by human service providers who are interested in prevention. The general conclusion that most mistreatment of the elderly is a function of the caretaker's being overburdened or isolated suggests that reducing the burden of providing care would reduce the likelihood of neglect or abuse.

The Michigan study and other research have identified many contributing causes of neglect and abuse. Inadequate health or knowledge of the caretaking adult, competing family needs, insufficient living space, or other problems of the care providers or recipients have been suggested. Although the research on the problem is insufficient, these observations are sufficiently consistent with the larger body of knowledge of the elderly and intergenerational relationships that such sources of stress and other problems are credible as causal factors of neglect or abuse (Brody, 1981; Weeks & Cueller, 1981; Hickey & Douglass, 1981; Smith & Bengtson, 1979). Virtually all financial stress or psychosocial stress, as noted in the studies above, are the central concerns of one or more types of service resource, be it a visiting nurse program, home heating cost assistance, or a friendly visiting program of volunteers. Although the majority of all service categories to the aging are underdeveloped in most communities, it is reasonable to examine existing programs regarding their potential role in prevention of mistreatment of dependent elderly.

The utilization of existing service options for prevention of mistreatment of the elderly is based on three consistent research findings. First, the manifestations of mistreatment are not equally prevalent and those forms most frequently encountered in the community are most probably caused by inadequate or inappropriate informal care circumstances or inept care givers. Physical abuse and active neglect, which are most likely to be caused by developmental or emotional problems of a caretaker or a pathological relationship between the givers and recipients of care, are apparently less prevalent than other manifestations. It is more feasible to accomplish prevention by improving the circumstances of domestic care and/or the competence of caregivers than by proactively diagnosing or intervening in situations which may be characterized by malicious behaviors of caretakers.

Second, the social gerontological literature, as succinctly stated by Brody has "systematically disproved the notion that contemporary families are alienated from the aged and do not take care of them as used to be the case in the 'good old days' " (Brody, 1981, p. 471). Yet the preparation of families for long term *family* care of an aged relative in terms of techniques of care, attitudes or expectations, or financial considerations is woefully inadequate (Treas, 1977; Weeks, 1981). Given that the majority of care of dependent elderly is provided by family members, the situations which lead to neglectful or abusive relationships may be modified by family support services which improve the circumstances of care for the elderly and prevent mistreatment. Better training and life span education, in combination with financial incentives for in-home family care of a dependent elder, can be expected to be cost-effective methods of preventing some forms of neglect and abuse.

Many cases of neglect or abuse which have been reported are caused by families who are stretched to a breaking point by not having any periodic relief from providing care. A respite from the responsibility and physical and emotional demands of providing care is critical for the maintenance of quality care and the prevention of neglect and abuse. This may be the most promising of all prevention activities because respite care also serves to meet many other desirable objectives regarding family relationships and the elderly.

Third, as highlighted by the O'Malley et al. study in Massachusetts and the Michigan study, different types of professionals have different probabilities of becoming aware of potentially abusive or neglectful situations before mistreatment has already taken place. Emergency room teams are unlikely, for instance, to be positioned to prevent neglect or abuse; their role is to appropriately treat the victims. Hospital based social services, however, have the responsibility to recognize the consequences of neglect and abuse and to initiate action to prevent the victim from being returned to a hazardous situation. Standardized case identification and referral procedures which exist for child neglect and abuse should be modified for aged victims in primary care settings.

Existing structures of public health and community mental health are well suited to identify potential and existing cases of neglect and abuse of the elderly. Public health nurses and visiting nurses become aware of home situations in which elderly people are dependent on care from relatives or friends. Often elderly patients are released from hospital care to family members. Social services already working with violent homes can become aware of vulnerable elderly who live in homes of neglected or abused children. Mental health counselors who learn of cases while working with other family members can initiate assistance to elderly victims. All of these community resources, however, must be educated about the nature of neglect and abuse of the elderly and must learn to anticipate cases as they now do for cases of child neglect and abuse. Professionals must also be free to act when action may challenge the confidential bond of professional and client/patient; thus, mandatory reporting laws are essential if secondary or tertiary prevention can be developed.

In order to understand the promise of prevention in the area of neglect and abuse of the elderly, it is first essential to understand the limitations of prevention oriented activities and programs. First, the elderly who are victims of neglect or abuse are usually competent adults and, while in need of help, have the right to refuse outside attention or intervention. Only in the most severe cases of purposive neglect and abuse should courts intervene to make victims wards of the court or to assign guardians. The rights and independence of victimized elderly should be protected as well as their immediate physical or emotional welfare. Second, primary prevention, at its most efficient level requires an operational knowledge of domestic caregiving situations which are at risk of becoming neglectful or abusive. After many years of research, target group analysis is imprecise for vulnerable children or spouses; limited empirical information offers very little target group guidance regarding vulnerable elderly. In the absence of indicators such as acute poverty, cries for help to an agency, or complaints from a neighbor or family member, prevention activities cannot anticipate situations in which caretakers are malicious and intentionally mistreating or exploiting the elders in their care. Secondary prevention is the best that can be expected in these circumstances.

Rather than outright violence or intentional neglect, the most prevalent forms of mistreatment of the elderly are caused by factors of poverty, poor health, or limited knowledge or skills of the caretakers in the home care situation. These factors are beyond the control of the victims or caretakers. In these cases the promise of prevention is very great. A network of health, social, and mental health field services exists which can be redirected. The majority of cases of mistreatment can be prevented if the human service systems direct their services toward the identification of families that have caregiving responsibilities to dependent elderly. The promise of prevention, therefore, is an improved quality of life for the dependent elderly and those who care for them, as well as the reduced incidence of mistreatment and fewer costly interventions for cases that are not prevented.

At the present time it is evident that there is an immediate need for additional research in the area of domestic neglect and abuse of the elderly. The research which has been conducted to date, particularly the Massachusetts and Michigan studies, should be replicated with probability samples which adequately reflect both the public and private service sectors. Detailed case studies of neglect and abuse must be conducted and rigorous evaluations should be expected of all public responses to this emerging problem. Evaluations of new programs, legislation, and the modification of existing outreach, casework, and treatment activities will give guidance to future efforts to deal with this emerging problem. Such guidance will be important in that the problem will probably increase as the population of frail elderly increases in the near future while alternatives to family care become increasingly insufficient.

REFERENCES

Block, M.R. & Sinnott, J.D. *The battered elder syndrome: An exploratory study.* Final Report to the U.S. Administration on Aging. The University of Maryland, Center on Aging, College Park, Maryland, 1979.

Brody, E. Women in the middle and family help to older people. *The Gerontologist,* 1981, *21,* 471-479.

Burston, G.R. Granny battering. *British Medical Journal,* September, 1975, 592.

Chiles, L. *Opening statement of the chairman.* Home Care Services for Older Americans: Planning for the Future. Hearings of the Special Committee on Aging, U.S. Senate, 96th Congress, USGPO 052-070-05146-9, Washington, D.C., 1979.

Cronin, R., & Allen, B. *The uses of reserch sponsored by the administration on aging. Case study no. 5: Maltreatment and abuse of the elderly.* Final Report to the U.S. Administration on Aging. AIR-82103-4182-RP, Gerontological Research Institute, Washington, D.C., 1982.

Douglass, R.L., Hickey, T., & Noel, C. *A study of maltreatment of the elderly and other vulnerable adults.* Final Report to the U.S. Administration on Aging and the Michigan Department of Social Services. The University of Michigan, Institute of Gerontology, Ann Arbor, Michigan, 1980.

Douglass, R.L., & Ruby-Douglass, P. Domestic neglect and abuse of the elderly. In R.G. Braen & C. Germaine-Warner (Eds.), *Management of the physically and emotionally abused.* San Diego: Capistrano Press, 1982.

Hickey, T., & Douglass, R.L. Neglect and abuse of older family members: Professional Perspectives and case experiences. *The Gerontologist,* 1981, *21,* 171-176.

Lau, E.A., & Kosberg, J.I. Abuse of the elderly by informal care providers. Paper presented at the 31st Annual Meeting of the Gerontological Society, Dallas, Texas, November 1978.

O'Malley H., Segars, H., Perez, R., Mitchell, V., & Kneupfel, G.M. *Elder abuse in Massachusetts.* Legal Research and Services for the Elderly, Boston, Massachusetts, 1979.

Rathbone-McCuan, E. Elderly victims of family violence and neglect. *Social Casework,* 1980, *61,* 296-305.

Rathbone-McCuan, E., & Hashimi, J. *Isolated elders.* Rockville, Maryland: Aspen Publications, 1982.

Select Committee on Aging, U.S. House of Representatives. *Elder abuse: The hidden problem* (96-222). Washington, D.C.: U.S. Government Printing Office, 1980a.

Select Committee on Aging, U.S. House of Representatives. *Domestic abuse of the elderly* (96-259). Washington, D.C.: U.S. Government Printing Office, 1980b.

Treas, J. Family support systems for the aged: Some social and demographic considerations. *The Gerontologist,* 1977, *17,* 486-491.

Weeks, J.R., & Cueller, J.B. The role of family members in the helping networks of older people. *The Gerontologist,* 1981, *21,* 388-401.